Addressing Obsessive-Compulsive Behavior in Autism with Functional Behavior-based CBT

W0018568

The Clinician's Manual and its accompanying workbook, *I Believe in Me, Not OCB!* are the first known manuals to combine cognitive behavioral therapy and applied behavior analysis to treat obsessive-compulsive behavior (OCB) in children and youth with autism. *The Clinician's Manual* serves as a practical guide for therapists, beginning with chapters that explain the theoretical underpinnings of OCBs, adaptations for autism, and guidance on clinical and functional behavioral assessment that are key to administering the nine treatment sessions that follow.

Our evidence-based treatment incorporates functional behavioral assessment, CBT skills training, caregiver coaching, and social skills activities in a nine-week progressive program. Caregiver and child report data inform progress throughout the program. Generalization and maintenance are promoted through weekly caregiver coaching modules. Treatment can be delivered in a group or individual format and focuses on reducing OCBs with the ultimate goal of increasing quality of life.

The manual provides all clinician, child, and caregiver instructions as well as materials to implement functional behavior-based CBT with precision. These manuals are a vital resource for clinicians working with autistic children and youth and their families.

Tricia Vause is a professor at Brock University and a registered clinical psychologist and behavior analyst. She is internationally recognized for her work in treating OCB in young people with autism.

Nicole Neil is the associate dean of research in the Faculty of Education at Western University. Her research and practice involve interdisciplinary approaches to applied behavior analysis.

Brianna M. Anderson is a PhD candidate at Brock University's child and youth studies department and has teaching, research, and clinical experience in applied behavior analysis, autism, and developmental disabilities.

Maurice A. Feldman is a professor emeritus at Brock University, registered clinical psychologist, and behavior analyst. He is internationally recognized for his research in parenting and developmental disabilities.

"These two manuals provide the best of both worlds of practice and research. They are the result of years of application and rigorous research into the effectiveness of a function-based approach to obsessive compulsive behavior. I highly recommend them to families, practitioners and researchers."

Peter Sturmey, *PhD*

"Based on over 20 years of research and clinical practice, this innovative program provides a practical, accessible approach to treating the obsessive-compulsive behaviours often seen in autistic (and other) children. Though flexible and individualized, it is very systematic and well-structured and is thoroughly grounded in theory and data. It could be billed as cognitive BEHAVIOUR therapy, with the solid theoretical base of Functional Behaviour Assessment providing an invaluable improvement on existing CBT methods."

Adrienne Perry, *PhD, C. Psych., RBA (Ont.), BCBA-D,*
Clinical Psychologist, Behaviour Analyst, Full Professor,
York University, Toronto, Canada

Addressing Obsessive-Compulsive Behavior in Autism with Functional Behavior-based CBT

A Clinician's Manual

Tricia Vause, Nicole Neil,
Brianna M. Anderson, and
Maurice A. Feldman

Illustrated by Pui-Lam Wong

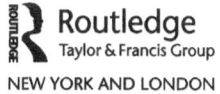

Routledge
Taylor & Francis Group

NEW YORK AND LONDON

Designed cover image: Cover illustration provided by Pui-Lam Wong

First published 2025
by Routledge
605 Third Avenue, New York, NY 10158

and by Routledge
4 Park Square, Milton Park, Abingdon, Oxon, OX14 4RN

Routledge is an imprint of the Taylor & Francis Group, an informa business

© 2025 Tricia Vause, Nicole Neil, Brianna M. Anderson, and
Maurice A. Feldman

Illustrations by Pui-Lam Wong

Library of Congress Cataloging-in-Publication Data
A catalog record for this book has been requested

ISBN: 978-1-032-72718-9 (hbk)
ISBN: 978-1-032-71230-7 (pbk)
ISBN: 978-1-003-41012-6 (ebk)

DOI: 10.4324/9781003410126

Typeset in Optima
by Apex CoVantage, LLC

Contents

Acknowledgments

The authors would like to sincerely acknowledge many sources of funding and support in the completion of this manual and the randomized controlled trial (RCT) that informed it.

Initial external funding was provided by the Children's Hospital of Eastern Ontario (CHEO) and Ontario's Ministry of Children and Youth Services. Subsequent external funding was provided by the Ontario Mental Health Foundation and Ontario's Ministry of Health and Long-Term Care. Internal funding was secured through grants obtained from Brock University (Faculty of Social Sciences and Office of Research Services) and Western University (Faculty of Education). Funding sources did not have a specific role in the RCT, nor in the content of this manual.

For both the Children's Workbook and Clinician's Manual, we adapted common elements from empirically supported cognitive behavior treatments for pediatric obsessive-compulsive behavior and anxiety (e.g., Franklin, Freeman & March, 2019; March & Mulle, 1998; Piacentini et al., 2007) and anxiety in autism (Reaven et al., 2012).

Dr. Tricia Vause would like to thank all of the undergraduate and graduate students whose work is reflected in this project, with a special thanks going to Dr. Heather Jaksic for her clinical contributions to the research that informed this manual.

Most importantly, we thank the participants and their caregivers for their generosity, dedication, and bravery in fighting obsessive-compulsive behaviors (OCBs). Their efforts allowed us to develop our knowledge in this area and disseminate our manualized treatment which we hope will reach many other children and youth struggling with OCBs.

Chapter 1

Obsessive-Compulsive Behavior in Autism

Introduction

Children with autism experience various challenges in social and communicative skills and display repetitive and restrictive behaviors (RRBs) that can often interfere with everyday life (DSM-5-TR; American Psychiatric Association [APA], 2022). Researchers have separated these behaviors into two broad subtypes:

- *Lower-order RRBs*: Motor and vocal stereotypy (e.g., repetitive, seemingly non-functional movements or vocalizations) and echolalia (e.g., repetition of sounds, words, or phrases spoken by someone else); and
- *Higher-order RRBs*: Circumscribed interests (e.g., intense, focused interests), insistence on sameness (e.g., completing routines in a specific way), compulsions (e.g., frequent handwashing to avoid contamination), and ritualistic behaviors (e.g., ordering and arranging; Bodfish et al., 2000; Guertin et al., 2022; Minshawi et al., 2014).

Higher-order RRBs are often topographically similar to symptoms characteristic of obsessive-compulsive disorder (OCD; DSM-5-TR; APA, 2022). Although not all higher-order RRBs are obsessive-compulsive behaviors, many are thought to reduce anxiety.

According to DSM 5-TR (APA, 2022), OCD is defined by the presence of intrusive thoughts, urges, and images that elicit anxiety and result in the overt presentation of ritualistic behaviors or covert display of mental acts (compulsions) that the person feels the need to perform to mitigate anxiety or in response to an established rule.

DOI: 10.4324/9781003410126-1

Why Do We Use the Term Obsessive-Compulsive Behavior (OCB)?

Autistic children often have trouble with introspection, perspective-taking, and describing thoughts and emotions that may drive the engagement of compulsions. It is often difficult to partial out what behaviors are "autism-related" and "OCD-related." Therefore, we use the term "obsessive-compulsive behavior" (OCB; Chok & Harper, 2016; Vause, Neil & Feldman, 2020).

Our approach is to probe for thoughts and physiological sensations associated with compulsions, but also, with the use of functional behavioral assessment, hypothesize function(s) of OCBs beyond anxiety reduction such as obtaining social attention from others or seeking automatic positive sensory stimulation. This treatment blends cognitive and behavioral principles and procedures to tackle the operant function(s) of OCBs that are reported as interfering to children and their family members, often daily, and that have a significant impact on their quality of life (Vause et al., 2017; Vause, Jaksic et al., 2020).

Functional Behavior-Based Cognitive Behavior Therapy (Fb-CBT)

We developed functional behavior-based cognitive behavior therapy (Fb-CBT) to address OCBs in autistic children. There is a well-established evidence base for the psychosocial treatment of anxiety disorders in autism. However, OCBs and the functional variables beyond anxiety reduction that may maintain this subset of behaviors have been largely overlooked in research and clinical arenas. Given our team's background in clinical psychology and applied behavior analysis (ABA), this treatment is a combination of two theoretical orientations: cognitive behavior therapy (CBT) and ABA (with function-based behavioral methodology).

Box 1.1   Functional Behavior-Based CBT

Functional behavior-based CBT (Fb-CBT) blends the well-established components of cognitive behavior therapy (CBT) with principles of applied behavior analysis (ABA) and functional behavioral assessment to address why an individual engages in individual OCBs.

Our Fb-CBT aims to tackle OCBs that interfere in areas including education, social, and everyday family functioning (Guertin et al., 2022; Vause, Jaksic et al., 2020). Throughout assessment and treatment, we first ask the child how OCBs affect them, and caregivers contribute by describing OCBs and helping to judge the interference these behaviors cause for the child and family members.

Fb-CBT consists of multiple components. Traditionally, treatments for both pediatric OCD and anxiety disorders have taken a predominantly CBT orientation (Ishikawa et al., 2007; Scarpa et al., 2016). The CBT portion of Fb-CBT is adapted from the solid evidence base in pediatrics (March & Mulle, 1998; Piacentini, Langley et al., 2007) and anxiety disorders in diverse populations such as autism (e.g., Wood et al., 2009; Reaven & Hepburn, 2003). Broadly speaking, CBT includes psychoeducation, cognitive and behavioral skills training, exposure, and response prevention (March & Mulle, 1998; Scarpa et al., 2016).

ABA principles (e.g., positive reinforcement and operant extinction) and procedures (e.g., behavior shaping and stimulus fading) are additive components of our treatment regimen that contribute to optimizing treatment outcomes for individual children. We use empirically based ABA functional behavior assessments and interventions as key assessment and treatment tools informed by the science of ABA.

Box 1.2   Functional Behavior Assessment

Functional behavioral assessment allows for the close examination of the operant functions of obsessive-compulsive behaviors (OCBs) that include anxiety reduction but also extend beyond anxiety to other potentially contributing variables (e.g., caregiver attention, internal sensory stimulation, escape from a task/activity).

Complexity of Treating OCBs in Autism

Operant functions should be examined with any clinical issue, but we feel they are particularly important given the complexity of assessing and treating OCBs in autism. This complexity stems from the overlapping symptom presentation of higher-order RRBs in autism and OCD, with these disorders showing similar phenotypic and genetic factors (Stone & Chen, 2016). This means that the behavioral topography may be similar and that a child may be predisposed to engage in these behaviors or that they run in families (Schnabel et al., 2020). For example, caregivers or siblings may engage in similar behaviors, or they may experience related challenges (e.g., social or generalized anxiety).

We mentioned earlier that given challenges in introspection and awareness of self and others, it is often difficult for children to vocally describe their obsessions, compulsions, and accompanying physiological sensations. *This is not just the case for autistic children!* In general, neurotypical school-age children often have difficulty communicating the thoughts and sensations that pair with their compulsions (APA, 2022).

Having partial or limited information about obsessions and compulsions often makes it challenging to discern the function(s) of OCBs, including anxiety reduction, making it difficult for a clinician to see the whole picture! In our experience, when discussing an OCB, school-age children may be able to describe the steps involved in the compulsion but get stuck when trying to talk about the obsession. Some common responses of children we routinely observe include "I just need to do it" or "I don't know." Sometimes, a child may offer a nonvocal response like putting a hat over their face. This makes it difficult for a clinician to determine whether the compulsion is completed to relieve anxiety/emotional distress, serves an alternative operant function (e.g., seeking caregiver attention, internal positive sensory stimulation), or both. Several suggestions on how to probe for more information are provided as you progress through the chapters of this clinician manual.

Obsessive-Compulsive Behaviors and Perceived Operant Functions

Let's look at Figure 1.1 to further examine perceived operant functions with OCD compulsions and higher-order RRBs. Figure 1.1 shows compulsions of OCD (left side) and higher-order RRBs (right side). Compulsions of OCD are driven by intrusive thoughts, urges, or images (e.g., worries about getting sick; images of imminent harm to self or others) that cause anxiety and unpleasant physiological responses (e.g., increased heart rate or labored breathing) for the child.

In clinical practice, we have worked with various presentations of OCB. We have worked with several children and youth who were afraid of something bad happening to themselves or others. For example, we treated a school-age child who frequently watched the changes in weather on social media and was afraid of rain, thunder, and other weather-related conditions placing a caregiver in danger. They engaged in several compulsions, including repeatedly asking for reassurance that the caregiver was safe when not present in the home, watching for the

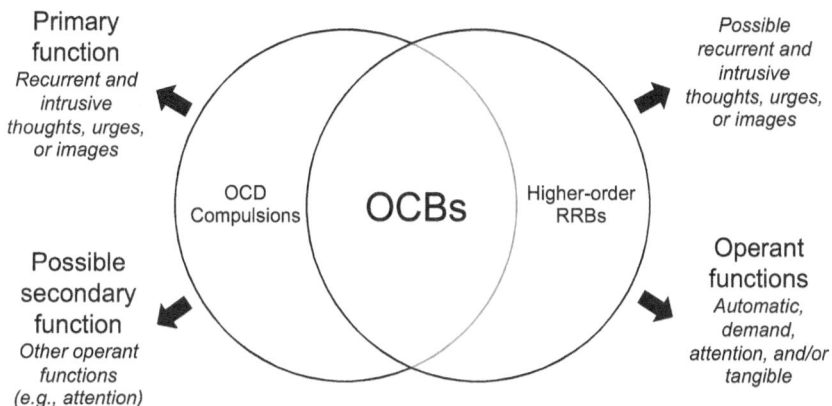

Primary function
Recurrent and intrusive thoughts, urges, or images

Possible secondary function
Other operant functions (e.g., attention)

OCD Compulsions

OCBs

Higher-order RRBs

Possible recurrent and intrusive thoughts, urges, or images

Operant functions
Automatic, demand, attention, and/or tangible

Figure 1.1   Operant function(s) and the overlapping nature of OCBs.

caregiver's car outside the home's front window, and repeatedly checking a weather app. These compulsions may also be maintained by secondary functions such as positive attention from others (e.g., an adult repeatedly saying, "Don't worry, your father will be home soon").

Similar to OCD, higher-order RRBs (right side) may also begin with a thought or unpleasant feeling that leads to the performance of a given behavior to reduce anxiety. For example, a child may feel uneasy if their caregiver takes an alternate route to school and may insist on the usual route to reduce an uneasy feeling or anxiety symptoms. However, other operant functions may be at work, such as a desire to take a similar route to view certain landmarks (automatic positive reinforcement) or passing by a fast-food restaurant to stop and order favorite items (access to a tangible). Given the difficulty in discerning function or the operation of multiple functions, we use the term obsessive-compulsive behavior, or OCB. Difficulties in articulating obsessions and other possible barriers, such as cognitive and linguistic challenges, may make it difficult to determine the relative contribution of identified functions of OCBs. To tackle each operating function properly, continuous assessment, modifications, and fine-tuning of the respective multicomponent intervention is often needed.

A Clinical Case Example From Our Research Lab

A functional behavior assessment may reveal an operant function quite quickly, or it may become more apparent as treatment progresses and the child can verbalize (in their chosen linguistic modality such as vocal

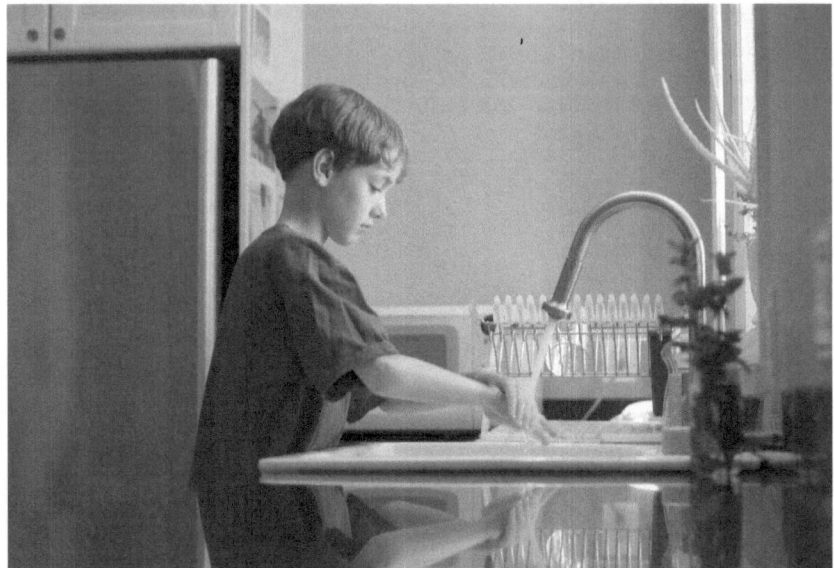

Figure 1.2 12-year-old Camden exhibits challenges with excessive handwashing.

language or an augmentative communication system) more information about a given OCB. For example, our research team treated Camden (a 12-year-old youth) for several months who engaged in repetitive hand-washing (compulsion). In the initial clinical intake, this school-age youth clearly discussed contamination-related worries and images of germs (obsessions) that resulted in the urge to hand-wash for long periods.

However, as treatment progressed over several weeks in our center and at home, other behavioral functions were revealed. They showed enjoyment (e.g., smiling, making vocal comments) regarding the feeling of the warm water contacting the hands, suggesting an automatic posi-tive sensory stimulation function for handwashing. In this case, a dual function was identified for this youth over time, and a multicomponent intervention was refined. The intervention accounted for the possible dual function and was brainstormed with the child and caregiver before being fully implemented. In addition to reducing overall handwashing duration, we equipped this youth with cognitive and behavioral strate-gies, including self-talk statements, such as "I can wash for one min-ute!" We implemented a functional replacement behavior involving accessing warm water (sensory stimulation) from a small indoor foun-tain. For detailed descriptions, refer to Chapter 3 of this manual and a peer-reviewed article from our research lab (Guertin et al., 2022).

Two Types of OCB

In addition to worrying that something bad may happen to themselves or others, OCD symptoms in children may also be maintained by a feeling that something is "not just right." March and Mulle (1998) and other colleagues discuss two types of OCD: worries about something bad happening to self or others (like contacting germs as discussed in our case example) or a persistent feeling of something not being right (e.g., feeling tension or tingling in a part of the body, or a repetitive thought of "I don't feel right"). A child may engage in an OCB (insisting on going the same route to school) to alleviate an uncomfortable bodily sensation/unpleasant feeling. However, the "not just right" feeling may also be accompanied by other functions such as automatic positive sensations (like in the case of Camden, who liked the warm feeling of water) or accessing caregiver attention and preferred items. For a clinician to optimize treatment outcomes, obtaining ongoing knowledge about individual function(s) maintaining an OCB is essential.

Why Does the Cycle of OCBs Continue and How Are They Maintained?

Refer to Figure 1.3 for the cycle of OCBs, incorporating both CBT and foundations of ABA. The figure illustrates the cycle of obsessions and compulsions. The top circle depicts obsessions (recurrent and intrusive thoughts, urges, or images; APA, 2022) that result in psychological distress (e.g., anxiety, fear) and associated physiological responses (e.g., increased heart rate, sweating). In behavior-analytic terms, these thoughts, the elicited distress, and the altering of physiology from internal and external stimuli may act as establishing operations (EOs). When speaking of an EO, the momentary value of reducing the distress or an unpleasant physiological response is increased, which results in an increased likelihood of a child performing a given compulsion. When a child performs a compulsion, there is a reduction in the child's distress. This temporary relief from the intrusive thought/physiological distress then evokes the cycle of automatic negative reinforcement, such that there is an increase in the likelihood that the child will engage in the compulsion again when encountering similar stimulus conditions (Miltenberger, 2005; Martin & Pear, 2024).

Recall Camden, who displayed excessive handwashing and discussed becoming upset because of thoughts and images of germs on

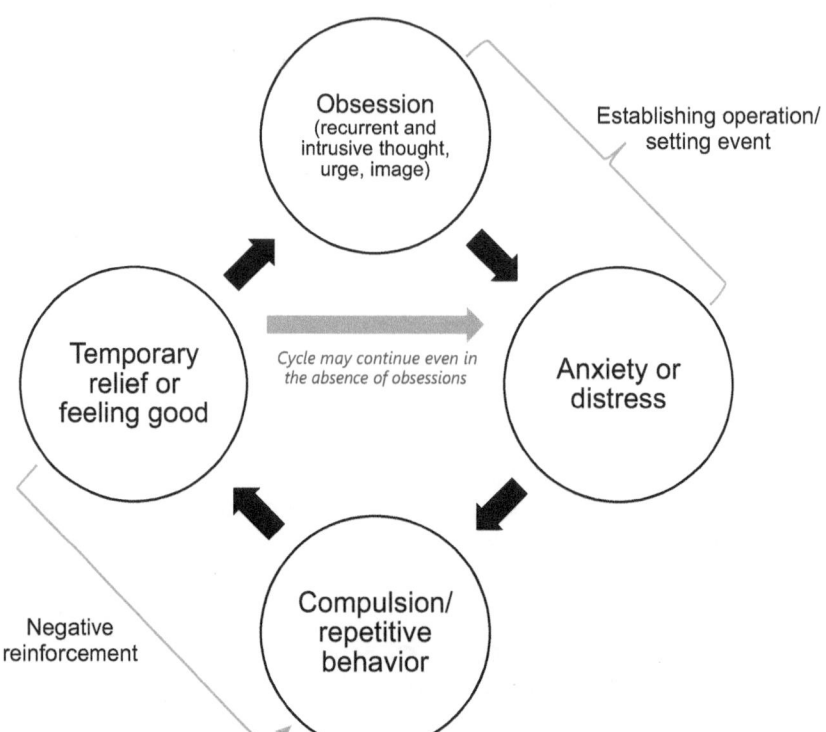

Figure 1.3 The OCB cycle.

his hands. This led to further contamination-related thoughts and distress about germs and contamination (the first two parts of the OCB Cycle are shown in Figure 1.3). The EO of distressing thoughts/sensations led to the strong desire to access a sink and wash his hands (the third part of the OCB Cycle; Figure 1.3), a desire he doesn't have when those distressing thoughts are not present. Because he knew washing his hands would alleviate this distress (the fourth part of the OCB Cycle; Figure 1.3), he accessed a sink and began excessively handwashing. As a result of the handwashing, he described feeling temporary relief from the distressing thoughts/sensations. In this case, handwashing reduced the EO and was negatively reinforced. In other words, given the relief he achieved by engaging in this behavior, he will be more likely to do it again when distressful thoughts and feelings arise (Guertin et al., 2022; Martin & Pear, 2024).

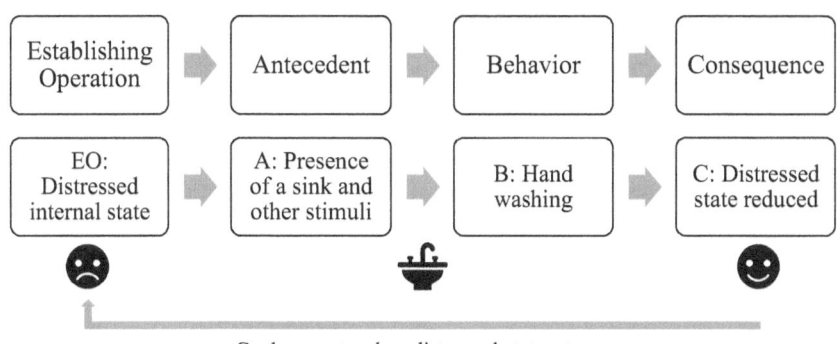

Figure 1.4 Illustrating the effect of the EO and negative reinforcement.

Tying It All Together: What Are We Doing Practically?

We have discussed the role of EOs and how OCBs are maintained over time. It is important to note that throughout a child's life, OCBs tend to wax and wane (March & Mulle, 1998). The tricky thing about OCBs is that one may go away, and another OCB may replace it. It may also be the case that individuals engage in different compulsions to relieve the same obsession. For example, we treated a school-age individual with contamination-related obsessions who was afraid of germs and getting sick. He engaged in behaviors of different contamination-related topographies (e.g., digging his fingernails in bars of soap and asking his mother to smell his fingers to obtain reassurance that they were clean). This extended to slamming his school locker a certain way to keep the "germs" out of food and tightly wrapping all food in plastic wrap that was in his lunch. For a more in-depth description, please see our publication by Vause et al. (2014). This is why it is important to adequately equip children and their caregivers with key treatment components they can use after treatment ends and as new OCBs arise or past OCBs re-emerge. Regarding re-emergence, our Fb-CBT sessions (outlined later in this clinician manual) focus on relapse prevention for multiple sessions at the end of treatment, which involves reviewing key treatment components and setting events; generalization to different people, stimuli, and settings; and practical tips on what to do when the same or different OCBs emerge.

An awareness of likely functions instead of solely relying on the topography of behavior is an essential part of our treatment strategy. For example, a child who is reluctant to communicate in social settings might avoid certain people or situations, cry, or exhibit physiological signs of anxiety or distress. In this case, identifying possible functions could help determine if treatment components should focus solely on anxiety/distress reduction (e.g., coping statements, gradual exposure, and response prevention) or if alternative function-adapted interventions also need to be implemented, such as providing alternative forms of sensory stimulation (as described for Camden). Functional communication training can be used to teach the child to access attention (e.g., "Please come here."), a desired item or activity ("May I please have a cookie?"), or escape a demand or unpleasant situation ("Could you help me?;" "I need a break!"; Carr & Durand, 1985).

For example, Maxim, an 8-year-old child who participated in our Fb-CBT, described an OCB that consisted of needing to print letters so they were "just right." As a result, he engaged in repetitive erasing and rewriting until he was satisfied with how they looked. In addition to other components, such as coping techniques, we put gradual exposure and response prevention in place, where he worked on being able to print the letters without erasing and fixing them. However, we also learned that pre-academic skills were challenging, and he had difficulty focusing on a task. He had a dual diagnosis of autism and attention

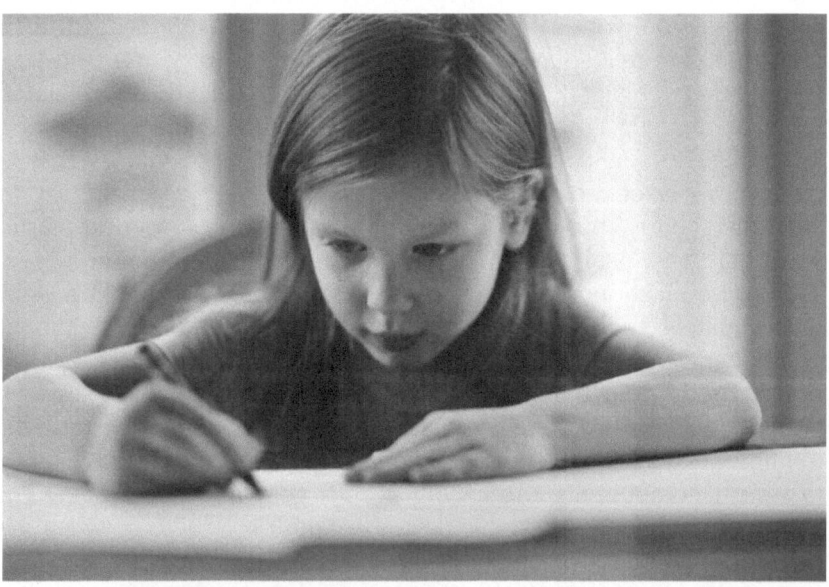

Figure 1.5 A client (Maxim) printing letters.

deficit hyperactivity disorder (APA, 2022). Specifically, he had trouble completing multiple pages of schoolwork and staying seated in his chair. Continuing to rewrite the same two sentences allowed him to escape completing the entire worksheet. To address the need to get out of his chair and take some time away from the task, we used functional communication training, which involved teaching him to vocalize when he needed to take a break and walk around the classroom or sit in an area with an exercise ball. This ultimately reduced the time he spent engaging in OCBs and increased the amount of schoolwork he could complete, even with incorporating these brief breaks.

Accordingly, Fb-CBT uses a multicomponent treatment to tackle all functional variables and gradually reduce OCBs. Given the multiple programming components and the expectations for the child and caregivers, we recommend working on a selective number of OCBs. To decrease stress, increase tolerability on the part of the child, and put reasonable expectations on children and their caregivers, we recommend tackling no more than two OCBs at a time.

About the Fb-CBT Manuals

Why Did We Develop These Manuals?

The Clinician Treatment Manual and the accompanying Children's Workbook were initially developed and empirically tested to fulfill an acknowledged clinical need. More than a couple of decades ago, in academic and clinical settings, the first author was increasingly asked, "How do you effectively assess and treat obsessive-compulsive behavior in children with autism?" In our experience, clinicians often said that they attempted various behavioral and psychological strategies and techniques but were unsuccessful in considerably decreasing symptoms/behaviors. However, given the interfering nature of OCBs, clinicians described themselves as feeling "stuck." They explained that they would attempt to interrupt the behavior and redirect the child to an alternative task but voiced that they needed additive or different components.

In many cases, the overlap between higher-order RRBs and behaviors characteristic of OCD makes assessment and clinical programming challenging. However, an approach that utilizes ABA (including functional behavioral assessment) and CBT components allows for a comprehensive assessment and treatment tailored to the young person's cognitive, developmental, and socio-cultural characteristics.

Who Can Deliver Fb-CBT?

These materials are aimed primarily at clinicians practicing with individuals with autism and related disabilities, including psychologists, applied behavior analysts, psychotherapists, counsellors, social workers, and medical professionals (e.g., general practitioners, psychiatrists). These books may be suitable for teachers, behavior therapists, educational assistants, learning resource teachers, special education and resource teachers, and caregivers (who have the training, acquire the necessary training, or are supervised to administer assessment and treatment components).

Targeted Age Group

Our Fb-CBT manualized treatment for OCB is designed for school-age children (ages 7 to 13 years). This age range is similar to the treatments evaluated through randomized controlled trial (RCT) studies for anxiety disorders in autism (e.g., 7 to 14 years, Reaven et al., 2012; 7 to 11 years, Wood et al., 2009). Given the differences in cognitive and socio-emotional development when comparing school-age children to adolescents, we followed the guidance of experts (e.g., Franklin et al., 2019; Reaven & Hepburn; Wood et al., 2009) when tailoring our material to school-age children. We aim to treat OCBs *before* they become more entrenched and more intractable to treatment (Boyd et al., 2012; Guertin et al., 2022). This manual can be used with children younger or older than this specified age range, but increased tailoring and personalization are often needed.

The Critical Role of the Caregiver in the Assessment and Treatment Process

The Clinician Manual and Children's Workbook are designed to be administered in a small group format (e.g., 3 or 4 learners: 2 therapists) or can be used for individual therapy. For both treatment modalities, it is ideal if the caregiver is present and plays a substantial role in assessment and treatment as both the coach and supporter. Of course, this varies from child to child. Still, school-age children often require varying levels of guidance and support within the session by their caregivers (e.g., assistance in describing an OCB or working through a treatment plan) and coaching in the home setting.

Prompting and support to design and engage in planned exposures in the home from caregivers allows for continuity of treatment in the home environment and sets the child up for success. Over time, children will become more independent in implementing treatment strategies, and the caregivers will gradually fade their assistance. **Caregiver data on OCBs** (see Chapter 2) is collected by the caregiver alongside the child report data to assess how the treatment is working and make decisions as a team as to whether to move on to a new OCB (as many children have multiple OCBs).

Adaptations Embedded into Fb-CBT

In Chapter 1, you will see a range of adaptations embedded into Fb-CBT. It is suggested that visuals are created to align with the client's preferences and support clients during various Fb-CBT components. For example, a fear thermometer is used to rate feelings of distress; however, to report the level of distress, children may respond to other rating systems such as a traffic light (red = difficulty in resisting compulsion; green = ease in resisting compulsion). Personalization of individual toolkits is essential. Some children benefit from visual prompts that are three-dimensional (e.g., a stress ball) or two-dimensional (cards with strategies written on them or textual prompts stored on an electronic device). For other children, visuals are not necessary, and reviewing strategies every week is sufficient. Visuals and different communication modalities (e.g., speaking vocally, drawing a picture, or using an augmentative communication device) can also be used to foster the social-communicative skills of each client.

Box 1.3   Choosing Your Battles

Talking about private or internal events, recalling past events, and using new reflection skills are cognitively demanding for children and may result in escape-related behavior. It is important to decide when to encourage children to persevere through fear-inducing situations and when to allow these "opting out" behaviors to occur. In other words, "choose your battles."

In our experience, children may prefer therapists and caregivers to scribe responses if writing is a non-preferred task. Documenting their responses should be the least effortful part of the process. Children are challenged with talking about private or internal events, recalling past events, and using new reflection skills. This is cognitively demanding, and if therapists or caregivers add on other complex tasks, such as writing, this may result in escape-related behavior or less engagement by the learner. We encourage therapists to reduce response effort in any way possible.

Throughout Fb-CBT sessions, children are offered choices, and therapists will become familiar with how material needs to be presented (e.g., the need for concrete information versus abstract information). Emotion cards (e.g., faces depicting various expressions) and role-playing can be used to support clients, and labeling the emotions of others and expressing how they feel in particular scenarios may supplement other communication modalities. Last, during the exposure and response prevention phase, reward charts are used where children are given a "visual" reward, such as a sticker or a checkmark, and a predetermined number of "visuals" are collected before receiving their reward. These adaptations and others are described as a part of assessment and treatment components. Appendix A highlights general adaptations for autism.

The Clinician's Manual

The Clinician's Manual serves as a practical guide for therapists to follow and begins with five key chapters that provide the necessary background and information that you will need to administer the nine treatment sessions that follow. In Chapter 1, you have already read about the theoretical underpinnings of OCBs and will soon be presented with a description of ABA and CBT components of Fb-CBT. Chapter 2 integrates clinical and behavioral assessment, and Chapter 3 outlines functional behavioral assessment and function-based intervention. Chapter 4 addresses social-communicative skills and suggests a progressive social skills hierarchy. For individual therapy, the social skills and games included in Chapter 4 may be implemented with the therapist, a caregiver, or just the child (at the therapist's discretion). We encourage flexibility on the part of therapists when selecting skills and games that they feel are relevant and additive components to the child's existing social-communicative repertoire. Finally, Chapter 5 briefly discusses considerations in running the nine treatment sessions.

Following these five chapters, the Clinician's Manual provides detailed information to guide the clinician through nine treatment sessions, each approximately two hours. The sessions are broken down into suggested time segments (e.g., 10 min., 25 min.). The length of each session is flexible, and variables should be considered such as the learner's motivation, degree of focus, ability to grasp information, and the complexity of OCBs. The outlines for Sessions 1 through 9 include how to arrange the environment, session materials, treatment components, a suggested order of components, and the approximate time to dedicate to each component. Caregiver modules are also included for each treatment session and focus on varying topics. Each child is equipped with the Children's Workbook that goes hand in hand with the nine treatment sessions and provides children with visuals and activities to complete the exercises provided in this manual.

This manualized treatment is designed so that each session builds on the next. Procedural and applied knowledge is scaffolded as well as expectations for caregivers to support implementation and increasing independence on the part of the child. Specifically, each session includes a review of the previous session, a report of OCB progress by the child (with the support of the caregiver and child's team), and then an introduction of new material and work on new OCBs. Before each session, a functional behavioral assessment (see Chapter 3) is completed by a therapist for each OCB to determine perceived functions.

Fb-CBT: CBT and ABA Treatment Components to Reduce OCBs

Like other CBT programs, our Fb-CBT includes psychoeducation, cognitive and behavioral skills training, exposure, and response prevention (March & Mulle, 1998; Scarpa et al., 2016). With this blended approach, we also explore perceived functions of OCBs and functional replacement behaviors to target the functions (e.g., receiving caregiver attention).

Psychoeducation and Stimulus Mapping

With psychoeducation, the therapist attempts to equip the child with sufficient knowledge, tailored to their cognitive developmental level, about both compulsions and obsessions and establish it within a bio-psycho-social framework (Taylor & Jang, 2011). This means discussing the fact that OCBs often run in families and are controlled by internal (psychological) thoughts and feelings and social variables such as stressors in one's environment and a wide range of family dynamics (Whitbourne, 2023). When conversing with children, we need to be mindful of their varying developmental abilities, cognitive barriers/strengths, and sociocultural background. These variables and others will impact the formation of a therapist's clinical framework and the lens they choose to take. It is important to be "developmentally" sensitive to the unique cognitive learning profiles of children and youth (Franklin et al., 2019). For example, some children function well with concrete information presented in "chunks" and examples that do not further perpetuate existing fears (Morris et al., 2021). As an adaptation, we gradually shape the child's knowledge of the term OCB by focusing mainly on compulsions (Session 1) and then talking more in-depth about obsessions in Session 2.

Psychoeducation involves referring to OCBs as neuro-behavioral (March & Mulle, 1998). This may be introduced briefly to the child if the terminology is too complex, and a more in-depth explanation may be given to their caregivers. It may also be saved for later in treatment when a child has a more thorough understanding of OCBs. For children, it is important to use visuals that they can relate to while explaining the "neuro-behavioral" nature of OCBs. For example, in our Fb-CBT, we present a set of visuals in Session 1 about contamination-related fears and associated compulsions with a central message of "It's not your fault. It just happens." This concept is illustrated in Figure 1.6, with an analogy of pins and needles. In other words, the brain sometimes sends incorrect messages to the body, causing actions or sensations that are not the child's fault; they just happen. Just like there are no "pins and needles" touching the child, there is not an imminent threat of danger from the thought of contamination.

Children who are aware of their obsessions and compulsions may have a learned history of blaming themselves or becoming frustrated when they feel the urge to perform these acts. Children may feel the need to attend immediately to emotional and physiological responses. Instead, we want to encourage them to view compulsions as incorrect messages from their brain that do not require their immediate action. OCBs are behaviors that come and go, and it is perfectly all right to let them do so. This cognitive strategy (discussed in more depth later in this chapter) is based on cultivating nonattachment (Franklin et al., 2019; March & Mulle, 1998) and dovetails nicely with narrative therapy work (e.g., Schwartz, 1997). **Externalizing OCBs** may involve viewing these behaviors as events that "come and go." Children are often taught to think of and call an OCB a nasty nickname (e.g., "Scram, you annoying creature!") or acknowledge OCB's presence (e.g., "Hi there, OCB" [nickname]). Children may choose to just sit with OCB or do something else that they prefer. Broadly speaking, you are teaching the child to accept that OCB is present, that it's OK they are there, and that OCB is not important and will eventually cease (like the pins and needles).

WHAT IS OBSESSIVE –
COMPULSIVE BEHAVIOR?

SOMETIMES YOUR BRAIN MAY SEND OUT WRONG MESSAGES. THIS IS CALLED OCB. OCB IS LIKE PINS AND NEEDLES. IT'S NOT YOUR FAULT AT ALL. IT JUST HAPPENS.

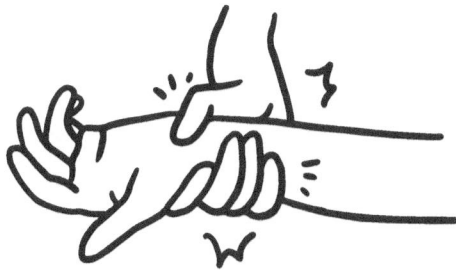

SOMETIMES WE TRY LOTS OF THINGS TO MAKE PINS AND NEEDLES GO AWAY BUT THEY JUST WON'T! HERE ARE SOME THINGS WE OFTEN TRY:

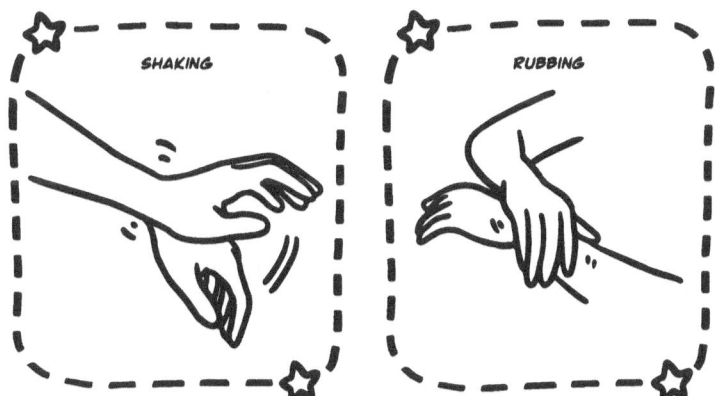

SHAKING

RUBBING

Figure 1.6 A metaphor describing OCBs and absolving the child from blame; it just happens (Children's Workbook).

We talk about the presence of these OCBs, which often feel like they are out of a child's control. Through our treatment and with the assistance of others, children can recognize their OCBs and feel energized to tackle them when they do come. In our experience, children like to use the words **battle** or **conquer**. In the words of March and Mulle (1998) and other experts in the field, children learn to "boss back OCB."

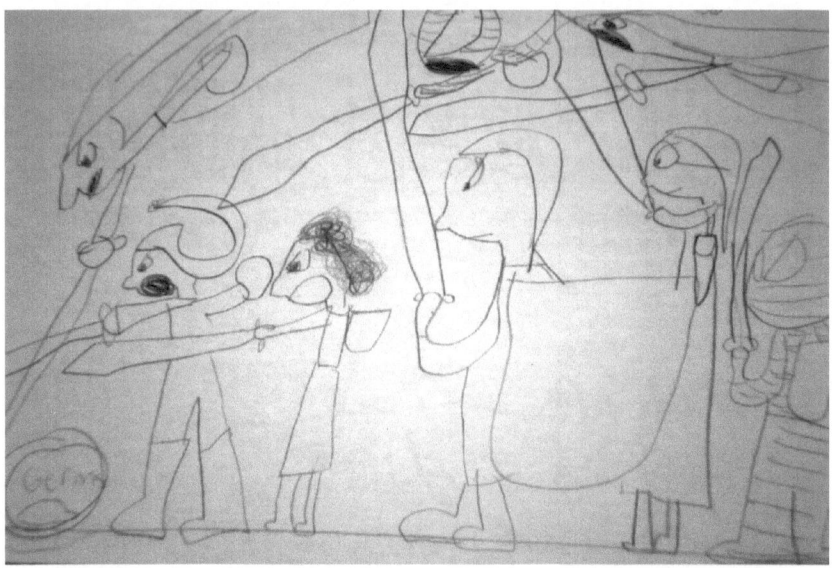

Figure 1.7 Drawing by a 10-year-old girl with contamination-related fears.

What child does not like being the boss? In our work with children over the years, they quite like being the boss and choosing who will be on their support team cheering them on and helping them tackle OCB!

During her participation in Fb-CBT, 10-year-old Sadie discussed being afraid of germs and insects in food items, such as fruit. As seen in the drawing in Figure 1.7, she drew herself as a large figure (in the center with a sword) surrounded by her support team. Therapists and her favorite characters (e.g., Zelda) and preoccupations (e.g., mummies) were part of the picture. Sadie explained that she designed the picture so that her team members were all pointing at the word germs (bottom left-hand corner). She further discussed that we were in battle and were equipped with shields and swords. Sadie was able to externalize the fears (germs) that drove her OCBs and see them as separate from herself.

Importance of Getting to Know Each Child

Autistic children may use stereotyped or idiosyncratic language or attempt to switch topics with a conversational partner to stereotyped interests or preoccupations. Perseverative or restricted interests (Klin et al., 2007; APA, 2022) may include topics, interests, and objects that occur among neurotypical children, such as computers and cars

(South et al., 2005), but can also include interests that are less common among neurotypical peers, such as washing machines or clocks (Wood, 2023). Perseverative interests are often a source of great pleasure for the child and a prime opportunity for shared enjoyment, communication exchanges, and teaching of various strategies. Therefore, we highly encourage therapists to embed unique interests into sessions to increase engagement, focus, and assist with rapport building (Harrop et al., 2019).

Concrete Learners and Adaptations

With young children who are neurotypical, explanations often need to be delivered in a concrete, straightforward manner. Traditionally, CBT incorporates Socratic questioning or open-ended questioning. For autistic individuals, this style of questioning may not evoke clear responses. Questions such as "Why did you do that?" may not result in coherent answers, and, therefore, clinicians might benefit from asking short and specific questions. Forced choice questioning may also be helpful (e.g., Do you arrange your items more at school or home?). Many autistic children also present with alexithymia, which is difficulty describing emotional experiences, especially subtle or complex emotions (Kinnaird et al., 2019). Fb-CBT provides visuals to assist children in discussing their worries (if present) and bodily sensations with the assistance of caregivers.

During the initial assessment, you could ask caregivers if their child is prone to behavioral outbursts and what triggers these outbursts so that you can be equipped with strategies to avoid or minimize behavioral episodes. With psychoeducation and other components, strategies may involve breaking tasks into smaller steps, interspersing preferred topics, and taking frequent breaks. Knowing each child's cognitive, developmental, and socio-emotional profile will help the therapist predict how to deliver treatment content and obtain optimal treatment outcomes. Remember the broad spectrum of concrete to abstract and that flexible learning styles are on a spectrum. Incorporating and attempting a variety of learning modalities and presentation of material may be beneficial.

Abstract, More Flexible Learners

For children who demonstrate the ability to engage in perspective-taking, demonstrate a deeper awareness of their behavior, and grasp abstract and complex concepts, it makes sense to have a more mature conversation with them. A clinician may need to attend to the words and gestures of the child closely and allow the child to lead the conversation and actively participate in the "unpacking" process. When conducting group therapy sessions, if interested, children who demonstrate these skills can be offered a leadership role or asked if they would feel comfortable modeling strategies for other children.

Importance of Child Voice

Listening to the child's voice is integral to the success of treatment (Reutebuch et al., 2015; Toussaint et al., 2016). Child's voice is the belief that all children have the right to express themselves in whatever way they can (e.g., using their voice, a communication device, gestures, facial expressions) and that their opinions matter when it comes to decisions that impact their lives (Twomey, 2020). For example, a child can choose a preferred item they want to work for during therapy or if they want to use a pencil or a crayon to fill out their workbook. Incorporating the child's voice into therapy can have many benefits, such as increasing child engagement (Lane et al., 2015), fostering independence (Unguru, 2011), and improving the child's self-worth (Anderson et al., accepted).

Considering the child's voice in individual and group therapy formats is particularly important. Some children may be more adept at voicing their opinions than others, but that doesn't make the quieter children's voices any less critical. You may consider different ways of soliciting each child's voice, such as providing opportunities to voice their opinions separately in a group environment or providing additional prompts in individual therapy. It is also important to recognize how a child's voice can manifest (e.g., verbal agreement, gestures, changes in body language). Not every child will be able to express themselves using words, so it is important to become familiar with each child's unique way of communicating. For example, a child may point to or move toward their preferred option when given a choice, or they may smile when presented with one choice and frown when presented with another (Anderson et al., accepted). Alternatively, a child may move away from an anxiety-inducing situation or begin to fidget when they are experiencing anxiety.

Box 1.4   Child Voice

Each child is unique, and just because they don't use their words doesn't mean they aren't using their "voice."

It is important to understand how anxiety can impact how children use their voices. Making important decisions or not being given enough time to make decisions can exacerbate the stress these children are already experiencing (Vella et al., 2018). Providing encouragement and reassurance (e.g., letting the child know they can take a break or change their mind), embedding coping techniques (e.g., closing their eyes, deep breathing), teaching positive self-talk, providing a small number of choices, and giving ample time to make decisions can decrease distress and make the process far more inviting.

Similar to Sadie and her fear of germs, other children we have observed respond well to taking control and giving OCBs multiple nicknames and extracting these OCBs from themselves so that they feel the OCBs are under their control, rather than the other way around. We want children to internalize this knowledge and have the confidence that they can learn to control these behaviors with the help of their support teams. Figure 1.8 shows examples of "Things I Can Do and Say to OCB" written by a child. The first entry referred to a rule of mixing the sequence of events rather than performing them in the same regimented fashion. The second entry is a "do" coping strategy, which was 30 seconds of meditation (instead of the OCB). Lastly, the child wrote a bossing back statement to OCB, "*Scram, you are power drunk!*"

In Fb-CBT, psychoeducation is paired with **stimulus mapping**, which involves a hands-on map (in the Children's Workbook) where children operationally define compulsions (and accompanying obsessions) and, with the assistance of a therapist and caregiver, establish a stimulus hierarchy of their OCBs. In the assessment phase of treatment, they are asked questions like, "What can you resist, and what does 'OCB' always make you have the need to do?" This allows children to better understand what OCBs they have control over and when they cannot resist performing the compulsion. In Treatment Session 2, children begin to place their compulsions into the appropriate zones: (a) OCB Zone, (b) OCB/Me Zone, and (c) Me Zone based on the degree to which they perceive they can resist the compulsion. More explicit instructions are explained in Session 2 of treatment.

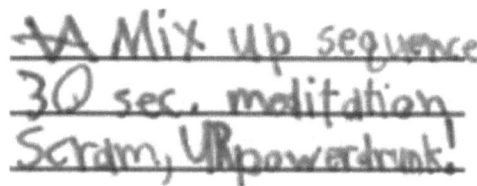

Figure 1.8 One child's quotes from our research.

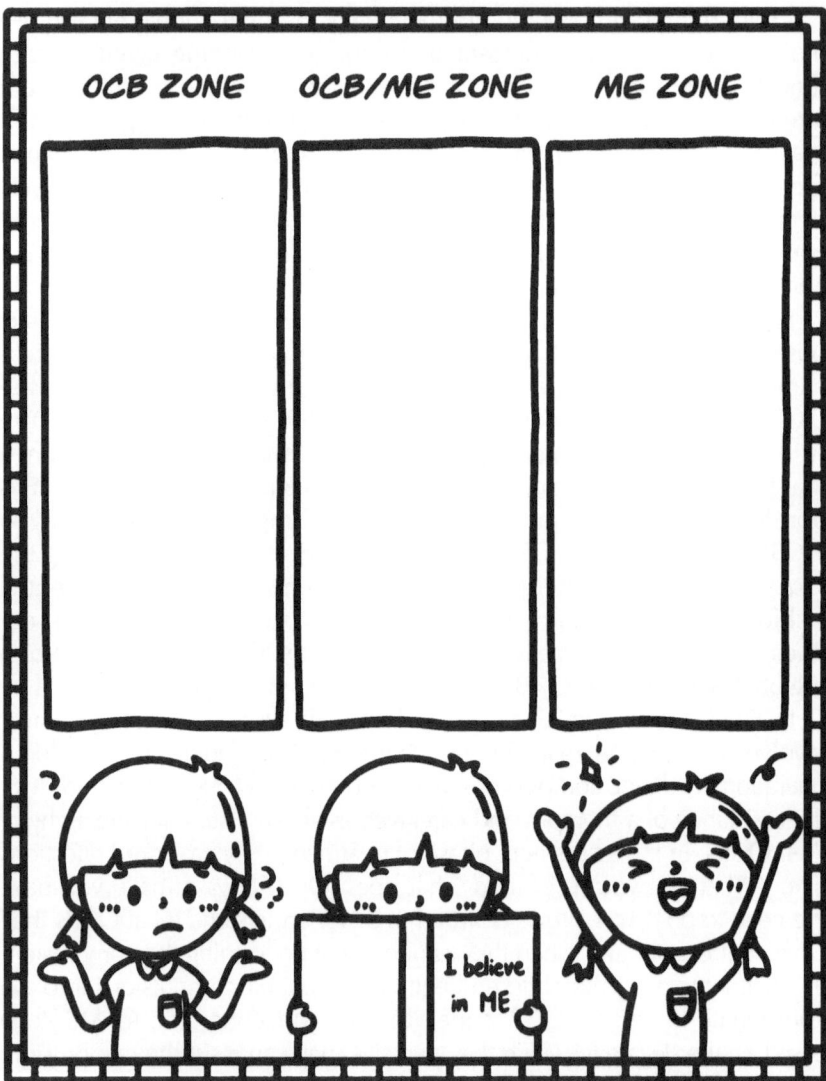

Figure 1.9 The stimulus map with the OCB, OCB/Me, and Me zones.

In each treatment session, the children revisit their stimulus map and move their sticky notes with listed compulsions to the right side as they gain control over OCB. The goal is to have as many compulsions as possible in the "ME area" (which means they can always resist the compulsion). This differs from child to child and with the complexity of the presenting compulsions (and obsessions).

Cognitive and Behavioral Skills Training

In Fb-CBT, children typically move between a series of cognitive and behavioral skills: (1) using coping tools in an attempt to alleviate anxiety/distress; cultivating non-attachment (described earlier); (2) engaging in functional replacement behaviors; (3) cognitive restructuring; and (4) self-talk.

1. Cultivating Nonattachment and Teaching Coping Techniques

In the previous section, we discussed teaching the child about externalizing OCB and that a child can separate it from self and "boss it back" or simply recognize its existence (March & Mulle, 1998). These statements are powerful for the child and show the recognition of OCB as external and something that can be worked on (March & Mulle, 1998; Franklin et al., 2019). In Fb-CBT, throughout sessions, children continue to generate bossing-back statements or review the ones they had previously come up with.

There are many cognitive and behavioral skills that can be placed in a child's personalized toolbox. From our experience with children, when programming for their first OCB, we explore many strategies, including those they prefer and have worked on with different behaviors and in varying contexts. As we progress through a child's stimulus hierarchy of OCBs, it is important to be aware of whether the child has tried to tackle OCBs and, if so, identify the child's favorite or "go to" strategies. In our experience, children prefer using similar strategies and tweaking them to the individual OCB. It is less response effort, has a proven working history, and is familiar to the child! We always begin by describing several replacement behaviors to children (e.g., engaging in social conversations with another person, deep breathing exercises, bossing back OCB with nasty nicknames, using positive self-statements), asking children which option(s) they think would work, and what they could see themselves doing. We then build on their ideas to create an individualized treatment regimen for each OCB.

Box 1.5 Replacement Behaviors

Replacement behaviors are more appropriate alternatives to distressing behaviors that need to be reduced (e.g., doing a deep breathing exercise to alleviate the distress caused by a contamination-related obsession rather than engaging in prolonged handwashing). Ideally, these behaviors would serve the same function as the compulsion, or in other words, allow the child to access the same outcome (e.g., alleviating distress or anxiety, accessing attention from others).

Figure 1.10 shows the workbook's My Toolbox activity that illustrates cognitive and behavioral skills examples. Beginning in Treatment Session 3, the My Toolbox pages appear weekly in Fb-CBT sessions as children begin actively working through individualized OCBs. This provides predictability, consistency, and prompts strategies they can choose from. Many traditional strategies targeted at anxiety reduction can be taught, including counting from 1–10 or engaging in relaxation techniques like muscle relaxation and diaphragmatic or belly breathing.

The pictures in the Children's Workbook may be used as prompts or ideas to explore "what works" for the child. In the workbook, we label these techniques as "My Toolbox." For example, the child may prefer belly breathing, counting, or they may want to "sit with OCB." Alternatively, the child may want to engage with OCB actively. For example, OCB may be represented by a stimulus such as Play-Doh that a child puts a large dent in with their hand and "bosses back."

To teach these skills, the therapist may want to engage in behavior skills training (Sarokoff & Sturmey, 2008) to demonstrate what the coping technique (e.g., breathing exercises; positive self-statements, such as "I know I can do it!") looks like and have the child *practice* to fine-tune the skill but also to test out whether it is a preferred technique. This also provides multiple opportunities for reinforcing the practice of the various techniques. As you can see, this is a mix of cognitive and behavioral techniques; some techniques are in the nonattachment realm (e.g., sitting with OCB and accepting their presence), and others are meant for anxiety reduction or emotional regulation (e.g., belly breathing).

Personalized coping strategies can help provide calming and soothing anxiety reduction properties and/or offer a replacement for the compulsion, where a child accepts OCB (e.g., accepting that their brain is

YOUR THERAPISTS WILL HELP YOU FILL YOUR TOOLBOX WITH
TECHNIQUES TO USE WHEN OCB COMES AROUND. PLACE A CHECK
MARK IN THE BOX AFTER YOU HAVE PRACTISED THE TECHNIQUE.

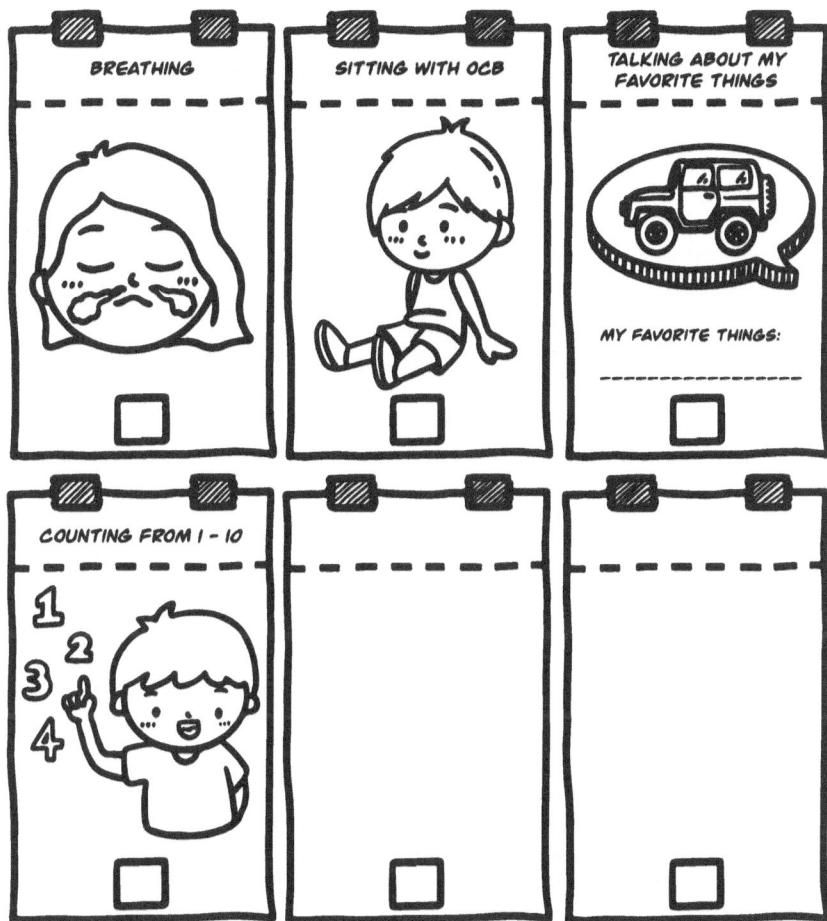

Figure 1.10 Coping tools and alternative activities that children can engage in
when OCBs arise (Children's Workbook).

sending them incorrect messages and that they can use certain strategies to disrupt these messages, such as using positive self-statements).
Children may use more active coping techniques (e.g., exercising or
muscle relaxation) or passive/nonattachment (e.g., reading a book). In
other words, children choose to detach from OCB and engage in an
alternative behavior. In most cases, treatment involves a combination of

cognitive and behavioral techniques or a combination of engagement in nonattachment and performing active cognitive behavioral skills.

2. Other Things I Need or Like: Addressing the "Whole" Child by Tackling Perceived Functions Beyond Anxiety

In Fb-CBT, "doing something else" is often linked to identified perceived functions. To make this understandable for the child, we use the general title of Other Things I Need or Like. For example, if a possible function is social attention from caregivers and specific social-communication skills are challenging, formalized programming such as functional communication training (Carr & Durand, 1985) may be put in place that involves teaching a child the various components of engaging in conversations or how to ask for and initiate a conversation to access social attention and increased involvement with a caregiver. If this is a "need" or identified likely function of the child, we want to ensure it is addressed. Another example might be fulfilling a sensory need with a replacement behavior, such as putting hands under a water fountain (in Camden's case) to feel the soothing nature of water instead of hand-washing, exercising, using sensory stimuli (e.g., small, soft toys), or programming times to experience a pleasant sensory sensation (such as sitting in a favorite seat). We want to address children's regulatory needs and emotional states so that each child feels balanced, comfortable, and safe.

The Children's Workbook has a diagram entitled "Other Things I Need or Like." This can serve as a helpful prompt for therapists/caregiver coaches to deliver the function-based intervention piece based on the functional behavior assessment. Children will sometimes add information in this section, but with some OCBs, this section may be left blank. In addition to acting as prompts for selecting coping techniques, these visual aids allow flexibility and the opportunity to brainstorm ideas with the child. At the same time, the caregiver and therapist also brainstorm ways to target likely OCB functions derived from the functional behavior assessment.

3. Thinking Differently About OCB: Cognitive Restructuring

If a child has the cognitive capacity and motivation to engage in cognitive restructuring of faulty thoughts and images, the therapist could attempt to utilize this cognitive technique. Negative or catastrophic thoughts and images often emerge because of the faulty perception of the probability that a catastrophic event will occur and/or that the child believes they are responsible for it and can prevent it from occurring by performing a compulsion. As March and Mulle (1998) point out, examining the probability of an event (e.g., a caregiver getting into a car accident) is often difficult for a school-age child to comprehend and having a diagnosis of autism adds additional challenges such as the ability to engage in abstract thinking. As a therapist, you may want to focus on the child's perceived role in an imagined event and their responsibility regarding the occurrence of this event. March and Mulle (1998) suggest a graph, such as a pie chart, to challenge a child's faulty thinking by brainstorming all the events that could be responsible for a feared event (e.g., a car accident). By doing so, conclusions are made regarding the extreme unlikeliness of the event being caused by the child.

In many cases, perceived responsibility can be challenging for school-age children. For example, a child may be afraid that their caregiver may encounter a car accident and need excessive and repeated reassurance from an adult (e.g., "Is Mom OK?"). Reviewing the reasons why car accidents occur (e.g., a car runs a red light, or a car may hit another when parked too close together) will help the child see that there are many reasons for events. In addition to examining "responsibility," you may attempt to visit "probability" on a basic level (e.g., you may review the unlikely chances of a car accident occurring in the first place). You may also review the proactive behaviors of the caregiver (e.g., wearing a seat belt, having a license to drive, and having a history of driving carefully).

A related example we encountered was an extensive bedtime routine, where the child needed to recite all the people, animals, situations, etc., in his life to keep them safe or needed a caregiver to do so. The child vocalized that something bad would happen if he did not engage in this reciting compulsion. In this case, the child perceived that it was his responsibility to protect people and things. Reviewing the reasons why people may not be safe (e.g., unhealthy eating habits, taking unnecessary risks) helped the child to see that there are many reasons why events happen and that the child had no influence over these events. Like the car accident example, we examined prosocial and safety behaviors that people in his life engaged in (e.g., eating healthy, exercising, sleeping, taking safety precautions in everyday life, safe driving habits). Last, we discussed "probability" on a basic level (e.g., a car accident that causes injury or death only happens rarely and most of the time because the driver is impaired or not acting safely). We discussed how prosocial and safe behaviors further reduce the odds of a catastrophic event.

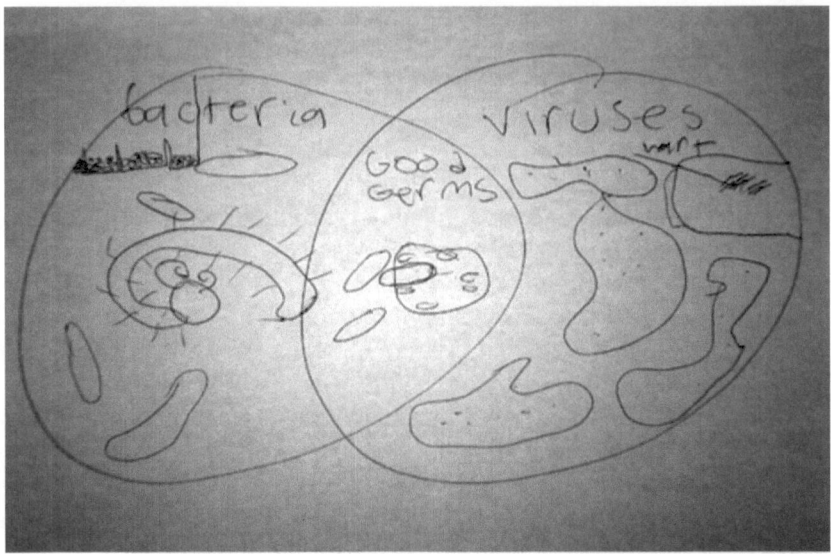

Figure 1.11 Child illustration of a cognitive restructuring exercise about germs.

As another example, Figure 1.11 shows a visual of Sadie's cognitive restructuring of germs with a drawing. Recall that Sadie drew a picture of herself and her support team fighting off germs. In this case, this young girl (with the help of her mother) read books on germs that her mother signed out from the library and, with this knowledge, could describe contamination fears in technical terms. Independently, she drew this Venn diagram depicting bacteria and viruses and vocally conveyed her understanding that some microbes are harmful and should be avoided. However, she also vocalized that some are safe and may even benefit our health. Sadie did not need examples of safe and unsafe exposures that may be necessary with a more concrete learner. We were able to have a conversation and restructure her thinking to appreciate the range of germs and the benefits of exposure in some circumstances.

4. Outsmarting OCB: Self-Talk

Self-talk that a child can use regularly can be generated from cognitive restructuring exercises. If cognitive restructuring is deemed difficult, the therapist could work on generating self-talk statements in the form of rules that contain pertinent information to challenge the targeted OCB. For example, let's refer to 12-year-old Camden, who engaged in handwashing for long periods. Cognitive restructuring was not utilized, but we devised OCB-specific rules such as "I can wash my hands for one minute." In this case, he established an initial rule (based on the recorded baseline being five minutes) and, in doing so, challenged OCB's rule of handwashing for five minutes. The rule may change as the child gets closer to the goal. In this case, "I can wash my hands for one minute" was the goal. If a child is not able to follow a rule that is specific to the OCB or if a specific cognitive barrier exists (e.g., challenges with receptive identification of time), the therapist may use protracted self-talk, "I can wash my hands for less time! Go away OCB!" and the caregiver may help the child keep track of duration.

Quite differently, for Sadie, who drew herself and her support team and was able to engage in cognitive restructuring around germs, we used the information jointly discussed and her Venn diagram to help her generate self-talk statements like "some germs boost your immune system." In this case, she engaged in auditory and visual processing of information. Self-statements may be internalized to a greater extent when containing child-generated information.

Last, how about OCBs maintained by a feeling that something is "not just right?" Consider the case of a 13-year-old girl named Molly, who said she experienced a disturbing tingling feeling in her hand that was only relieved by slamming the basement door three times. We were able to engage in cognitive restructuring about the irrationality of the connection between the tension in her hand and performing the compulsion. From there, she developed related self-statements such as, "I don't need to slam the door. The weird feeling in my hand will go away."

The Cognitive Behavioral Skills Template

In our research and clinical work, we encourage therapists to devise a preliminary plan before each therapy session (beginning in Session 3) using our Cognitive Behavioral Skills Template. Often, it is difficult to think on the spot, so our therapists prepared several helpful strategies in advance (e.g., social stories, visuals, "chunking" material, teaching discrimination between "good" and "bad" or "safe" and "unsafe"). A therapist handout to assist with pre-planning and outlining individualized treatment components is included in Treatment Session 2.

Gradual Exposure and Response Prevention

Exposure and response prevention (E/RP) is the process by which an individual is exposed to stimuli that trigger anxiety or distress and refrain from engaging in the compulsion. For OCBs, a common way this can be accomplished is by gradually "breaking the chain" (March & Mulle, 1998). In doing so, you can use different types of behavioral dimensions such as duration, frequency, latency, topography, and/or intensity/force of a response (Martin & Pear, 2024).

Let's review some of the cases described earlier. For example, in Camden's 5-minute handwashing, the behavior was initially set to 4 minutes. Through self-talk and other strategies, Camden had a final rule: "I can handwash for one minute!" In contrast, in the case of 10-year-old Sadie who exhibited contamination-related behavior related to germs, with one behavior in her stimulus class that involved avoiding touching and eating fruit for fear it contained germs and insects, she gradually increased the frequency of touching and then eating one kind of fruit; throughout programming, we expanded her diet to include a variety of fruits.

This is depicted in the March and Mulle (1998) manual and, in our experience, is a key piece for consideration when programming between and across OCBs. In the two cases of contamination-related behavior, the dimensions used made sense for the topographies of behavior, but others could have been chosen. Table 1.1 shows examples of common OCBs we have treated in our RCT research (Jaksic et al., 2018), related dimensions, goals, and specific examples.

Table 1.1 shows two dimensions that may be considered for repetitively asking for reassurance. This often depends on data collection feasibility, behavior frequency, etc. In another example regarding the use of latency to increase flexibility with lining up stuffed animals, there may be an initial program to target flexibility with stuffed animals and then a secondary component to work on eliminating stuffed animals from the line-up (see Table 1.1 for further details). Last, in the case of behaviors maintained by sensory properties and children satisfying regulatory states, the goal may not be to decrease the behavior to zero levels, but instead, to maintain it on a reasonable variable schedule (or the child can variably access it but not to the point that it becomes excessive).

Why Is Gradual Exposure Often Necessary?

Our RCT (Vause, Jaksic et al., 2020) and clinical experience in working with autistic children with OCBs, show that gradual exposure leads to increasing child motivation in attempting exposures and maintenance of OCB absence over time. In behavioral terms, we are gradually shaping the final desired behavior until the OCB no longer occurs or is no longer interfering with everyday life (Martin & Pear, 2024). The

Table 1.1 Examples of OCBs dimensions and goals

OCB	Measurement Dimension	Goal	Example
Handwashing or Showering for Long Periods	Duration	Gradually decrease the duration of handwashing to the target time.	*Beginning*: 8 minutes *Terminal*: 1 minute
Handwashing and Hand Sanitizing Several Times a Day	Frequency	Gradually decrease the frequency of the related compulsions to a target number.	*Beginning*: 10 times (both behaviors together). *Terminal*: 4 times a day of either behavior.
Repetitive Asking for Reassurance When Caregiver Is Not Home	Per Opportunity	Collect per opportunity data when the stimulus (caregiver being away) occurs	*Beginning*: Repetitive asking on every occasion of the caregiver not being home from work for a 5-day work week. *Terminal*: Asking occasionally when the caregiver will be home (1 or 2 times) during a 5-day work week. In some cases, frequency data may give a more accurate picture.
Lining Up Stuffed Animals in a Row	Latency	Have the child wait for progressively longer periods of time before moving the stuffed animals back to their original position	*Beginning*: 1 second. *Terminal*: The stuffed animal can be left in a different position. This would be repeated with different stuffed animals until the child is flexible with moving and leaving many items. A secondary component may be decreasing the number of stuffed animals in cases where they are interfering (such as 100 stuffed animals on bed).

(Continued)

Table 1.1 (Continued)

OCB	Measurement Dimension	Goal	Example
Slamming a Door with Palm of Hand	Intensity or Force	Decrease the force being applied	*Beginning*: Excessively loud sound of door closing. *Terminal*: Typical noise produced by door closing.
Morning Routine with Several Steps that Child Insists on Performing in a Predetermined Order	Topography	Remove one step or the child changes the routine in some manner	*Beginning*: All steps of routine done in same order. *Terminal*: Steps can be done in a flexible order. Irrelevant steps removed. Negotiation with the child regarding necessary steps and steps to eliminate or change order.
Sitting in the Same Seat	Frequency	Decrease the number of times a child sits in "chosen seat"	*Beginning*: Sits in chosen seat every time. *Terminal*: Is flexible in sitting in different seats but still gets to access chosen seat on occasion.

shaping process involves gradually introducing the child to distressing triggers while the child resists engaging in the OCB. According to the two-factor theory, this means the child is not only no longer performing the compulsions; they are also no longer feeling anxious or distressed when confronted with previously anxiety-provoking triggers (Guertin et al., 2022). Ample reinforcement is provided as the child successfully encounters triggers without engaging in OCBs. Despite exposure to triggers and stimuli in the environment (e.g., the kitchen sink), OCBs are reduced to near zero levels (e.g., handwashing for one minute). Reinforcement is systematically thinned until only naturalistic reinforcers are provided (i.e., reinforcement that matches what the child would otherwise receive in everyday life such as intermittent caregiver praise).

There are several reasons why offering gradual exposures makes sense. First, we want children to follow through! It also considers the child's voice (Twomey, 2020). This allows the therapist to offer the child an opportunity to have some autonomy in what they feel comfortable doing and to participate in the problem-solving towards a set of small goals or steps to achieve the final desired behavior. Breaking the OCB down into smaller goals may also help them to understand the OCB (and chain of behaviors). Second, breaking things down will likely increase the likelihood of children being successful in completing exposures (using their cognitive behavioral skills training) and using their coping techniques allows the child multiple instances of seeing that nothing bad happens when exposed to the anxiety-eliciting stimulus without fully engaging in the OCB (Pavlovian extinction). Frequent daily reinforcement should be provided for engaging in alternative behaviors. These experiences likely contribute to the gradual minimization of the OCB. The child will continue to be motivated to "fight" OCB and work through the hierarchy (typically starting with OCBs they have some control over and moving to highly resistant OCBs). Third, this is a unique and diverse population with many children working on other challenges such as social-communication issues, adaptive skills deficits, challenging behaviors, and perhaps other related mental health issues. We want to expose the child without overwhelming them (and family support members) or detract from therapeutic successes in other areas. Last, it is often a stressful experience for the caregiver to see their child experiencing symptoms of anxiety; gradual exposure allows for small successes with *some* mild anxiety leading in many cases to the elimination of OCBs.

Having highlighted the benefits of gradual exposure, it is important to consider time and resources. Using a gradual approach often takes longer. Also, it has the potential risk of lingering compulsions (e.g., the child gets stuck at washing hands for four minutes). The clinician must keep a close watch on whether any lingering compulsions arise. For example, a child may have an OCB of a rigid routine, and by eliminating a few steps, you have created a secondary rigid routine. It is also possible that the child does not experience sufficient anxiety with the gradual nature and habituation does not occur. However, in our experience and evaluating Fb-CBT with our RCT (Vause, Jaksic et al., 2020), children report feeling some anxiety during gradual exposures and use their recently acquired cognitive behavioral skills to help them resist performing the compulsion. Over time, the OCB is moved to the "Me Zone" on their stimulus map where the child feels they have full control of their compulsions.

When Is Flooding Appropriate and Preferred by Some Children?

Flooding is "a method of extinguishing fear by exposure to the feared stimulus intensely for an extended period" (Martin & Pear, 2024, pp. 288–289). We previously discussed 13-year-old Molly, who exhibited a "not just right" behavior of a disturbing tingling feeling in her hand and the belief that this sensation would cease if she slammed the door three times. After engaging in cognitive restructuring and discussing different options, she voiced that she preferred to tackle this OCB by attempting to eliminate it immediately. In this case, the starting behavior (or baseline data) suggested slamming the door three times, and she said she would work on "closing the door normally" just once. She modeled what this would look and sound like. She attempted this and was successful on the first attempt; many months later, this behavior had not returned. It is the clinician's hypothesis that after understanding the irrationality of a connection between her tingly hand and the door slamming a certain number of times, she opted to fully eliminate this behavior on her first attempt.

ABA Treatment Components

Functional Behavioral Assessment

The importance of considering functional variables is discussed throughout this chapter. Chapter 3 guides you through conducting a functional behavioral assessment (e.g., caregiver interview and narrative recording of behaviors). This is key to designing an intervention that tackles anxiety and other perceived functions (e.g., social attention) of OCBs and adapting the intervention as necessary. Therapists with advanced knowledge in functional behavior assessment may choose to conduct functional analyses (Hanley et al., 2014) that offer more substantial experimental control and confidence in the function maintaining the OCB.

ABA Principles and Procedures Are Central to Fb-CBT

Principles and procedures based on the science of ABA are embedded throughout Fb-CBT. Figure 1.12 shows a worksheet called "Stepping It Up: Completing My Exposures." Several ABA-based components are embedded in this activity as prompts such as (a) setting goals for an OCB exposure, (b) the opportunity to check a box if the child met their goal, (c) coloring in circles when using their coping techniques, and (d) a line

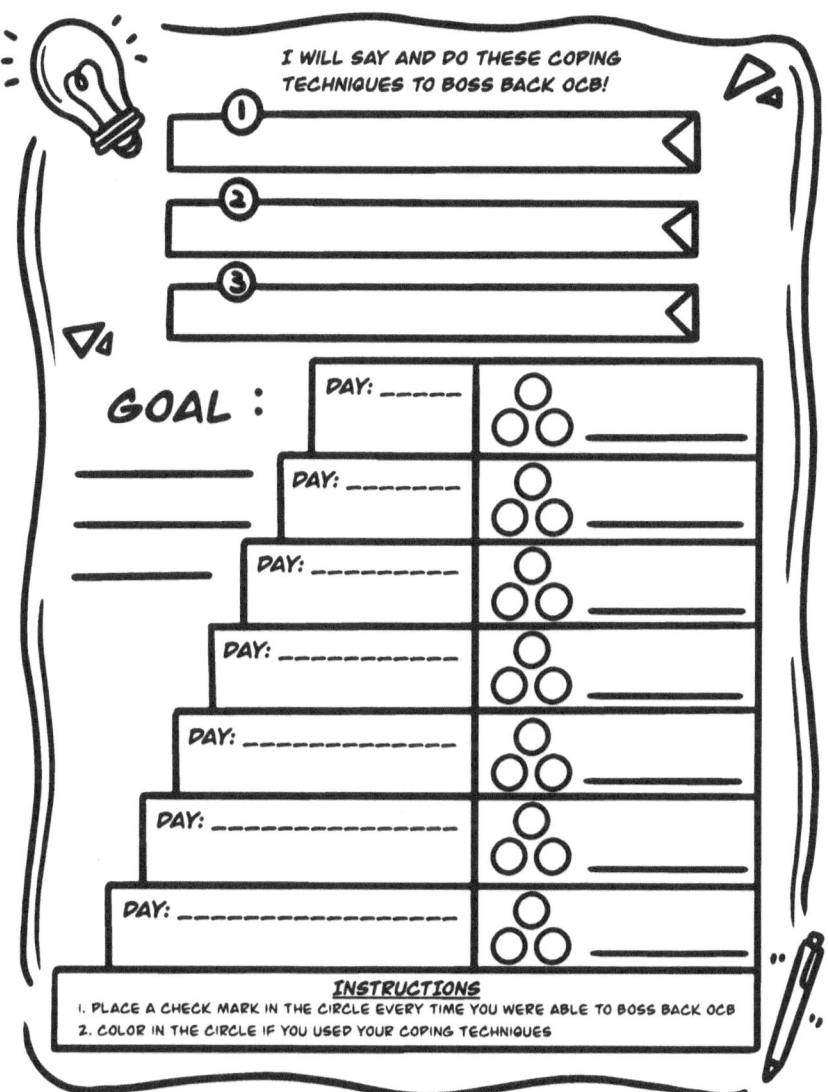

I WILL SAY AND DO THESE COPING
TECHNIQUES TO BOSS BACK OCB!

①
②
③

GOAL :

DAY: _____
DAY: _____
DAY: _____
DAY: _____
DAY: _____
DAY: _____
DAY: _____

INSTRUCTIONS
1. PLACE A CHECK MARK IN THE CIRCLE EVERY TIME YOU WERE ABLE TO BOSS BACK OCB
2. COLOR IN THE CIRCLE IF YOU USED YOUR COPING TECHNIQUES

Figure 1.12 Exposure/Response prevention activity (Children's Workbook).

to write in reinforcers/preferred items for completing each goal (Martin & Pear, 2024). We gradually shape the behavior with graduated exposure until the final desired behavior is present. Also, operational definitions are developed for each OCB that often involve *chaining* components together and gradually "breaking the chain" (March & Mulle, 1998).

In this chapter, the principle of positive reinforcement is discussed many times. Often, children with and without autism need frequent positive reinforcement to build skills. OCBs are maintained by strong negative reinforcement (anxiety reduction) and perhaps other reinforcing consequences. Therefore, children often are reluctant to stop OCBs on their own. Programmed reinforcement supports the child in participating in therapy, promoting prosocial behavior, and resisting performing a compulsion. There is substantial research establishing the effectiveness of token systems in increasing skills among children with autism (National Autism Center, 2015). Throughout Fb-CBT sessions, a token reinforcement system is used. Group participation decorum rules are explicitly stated in Treatment Session 1, including using appropriate volume and respecting others' personal space. Demonstration of prosocial behavior results in tokens (or something preferred, like a sticker) exchanged for individualized preferred items (a backup reinforcer) at the end of sessions.

In the home, caregivers reward the child for completing practice exposures with checkmarks that can be exchanged for preferred items. The child and caregiver brainstorm these items, which can be tangible items (e.g., increased access to a tablet to play games or watch videos), extra time doing something fun with a caregiver, choosing the restaurant for a family meal, staying up later at bedtime, etc. During sessions, the list of possible backup reinforcers is revisited weekly as the child's preferences may change. Also, the token system offers the opportunity to discuss a topic that is often pleasant for children and where they can negotiate and have a voice in "what they would like to work for." Caregivers may need coaching to provide differential reinforcement (e.g., more checkmarks are given for accomplishing more challenging goals, fewer for easy goals). Caregivers may also need help determining how much preferred items cost, with more expensive or highly preferred items (big rewards) costing more checkmarks than less expensive and readily available items (small rewards). See Figure 1.13 for a visual activity for writing or drawing big and small reinforcers. For further information on using token systems in session and at home, please refer to Treatment Session 1. For a sample reinforcer checklist, See Appendix B.

In our treatment, children typically share their experiences working on the targeted OCB at the beginning of the session. They continue to work on the present OCB and record their exposures (even if they are close to resisting it most of the time). Then, when the OCB is at a desired level, we want to ensure the maintenance of OCBs at this level,

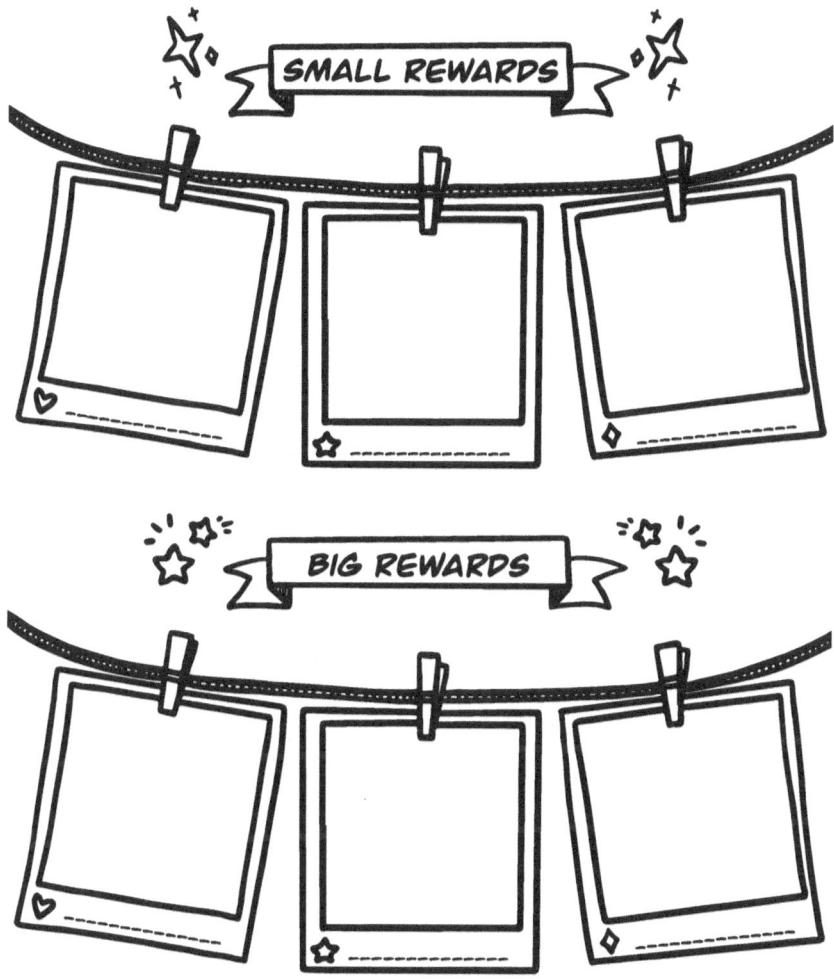

Figure 1.13 An example of small and big reinforcers.

especially when the child continues to be exposed to stimuli/triggers even if the obsession/distress is absent. This is important because OCBs tend to wax and wane, and we want to ensure that OCB absence is maintained after treatment ends. We also fade out the artificial reinforcers when OCBs dissipate and replace them with natural reinforcers (e.g., caregiver recognition) that can maintain the absence of previously targeted OCBs. For example, for the 10-year-old who began to eat fruit and fought off the urge to avoid the food (given thoughts of contamination), the caregiver may say, "I like how you're eating fruit and getting that Vitamin C!" Our stimulus map (see Children's Workbook) often fosters self-praise statements (e.g., the child feels proud of their accomplishments in fighting OCBs) when an OCB is moved to the "Me Zone."

Weekly Caregiver Coaching Modules: Scaffolding of Treatment Component Skills

Caregiver involvement is an integral part of the treatment. Specifically, caregivers engage in intensive caregiver coaching sessions of approximately 25 minutes or more per session. Training is conducted systematically to gradually shape caregivers' ABA and CBT knowledge and skills through carefully laid out caregiver modules.

The caregiver coaching modules progress as follows: (a) discussion of OCB etiology and maintenance to develop conceptual understanding, (b) hands-on training on functional behavioral assessment and intervention for their child's OCBs, (c) individualized cognitive and behavioral skills training, (d) how to design and conduct exposure and response prevention with their child's existing OCBs, (e) fading artificial reinforcement to reliance on natural reinforcers only, and (f) relapse prevention.

An empirically supported coaching method is **behavioral skills training** (Anderson et al., 2023; Parsons et al., 2012; Sarokoff & Sturmey, 2008). This method consists of four steps: instruction, modeling, rehearsal, and feedback (see Figure 1.14).

Fb-CBT has a systematic lesson plan for each module using behavioral skills training for skills caregivers can learn in session and implement at home. Regarding caregiver coaching, we use a most-to-least prompting model (Martin & Pear, 2024) over treatment sessions, where caregivers learn the treatment components in caregiver modules. Then the therapist gradually fades their presence while the caregiver (and child) assume a more significant role in developing treatment plans, choosing reinforcers, etc. This transfer of support (i.e., therapist to caregiver/child) is individualized to the caregiver-child dyad.

Group and Individual Social-Communicative Skills

Social skills are a critical component of child development, and yet they are a core challenge for many autistic individuals. Drawing on CBT- and ABA-based social skills research (Steinbrenner et al., 2020) and neurodiversity-affirming teaching approaches (Mathur et al., 2024), our manual includes activities to help autistic individuals build social-communicative skills. Week-by-week, activities gradually increase in

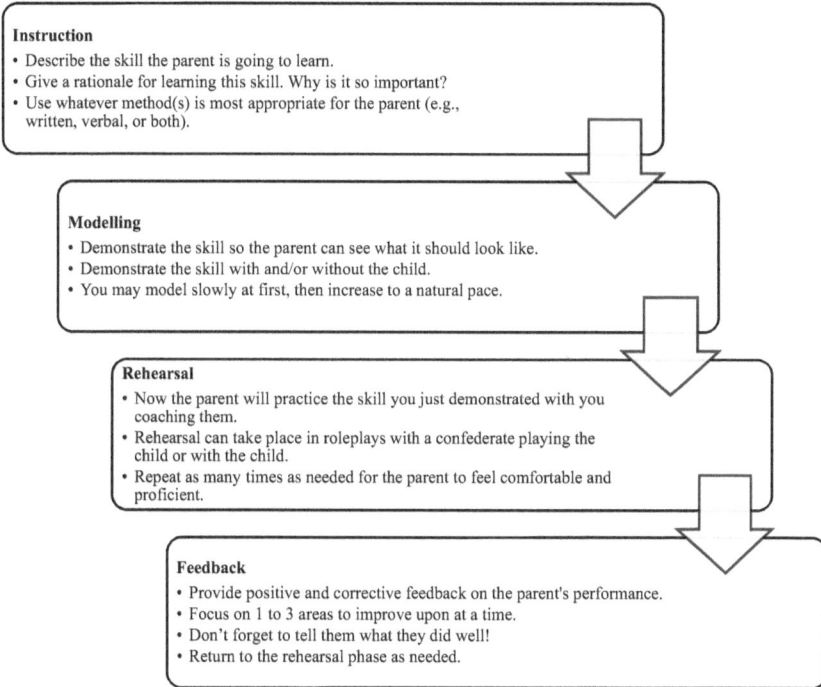

Instruction
- Describe the skill the parent is going to learn.
- Give a rationale for learning this skill. Why is it so important?
- Use whatever method(s) is most appropriate for the parent (e.g., written, verbal, or both).

Modelling
- Demonstrate the skill so the parent can see what it should look like.
- Demonstrate the skill with and/or without the child.
- You may model slowly at first, then increase to a natural pace.

Rehearsal
- Now the parent will practice the skill you just demonstrated with you coaching them.
- Rehearsal can take place in roleplays with a confederate playing the child or with the child.
- Repeat as many times as needed for the parent to feel comfortable and proficient.

Feedback
- Provide positive and corrective feedback on the parent's performance.
- Focus on 1 to 3 areas to improve upon at a time.
- Don't forget to tell them what they did well!
- Return to the rehearsal phase as needed.

Figure 1.14 Behavioral skills training coaching model (Parsons et al., 2012; Sarokoff & Sturmey, 2008).

complexity, also known as scaffolding. This progressive format allows children to practice various social skills without the added frustration. More details on our social skills activities can be found in Chapter 4.

Accompanying Children's Workbook

The accompanying Children's Workbook is used in all treatment sessions, and the child brings it home each week to review strategies, practice, and record in-home exposures. As we know, the structured nature of CBT can be supportive for children with autism. It provides structured sessions, with predictable activities each week. Each session has a visual schedule that indicates the order of events, and children can mark the completion of each activity. Treatment components also occur in roughly the same order each week. Although the schedule is predictable, we gradually encourage work on flexibility by introducing new OCBs with individualized adaptations (e.g., use of visuals and attempting different cognitive techniques). The workbook contains hands-on exercises to complete in session and worksheets to collect data at home. In the workbook, children can track progress over time (with the stimulus map) and refer to visual material of each week's concepts. When the nine sessions are complete, children are encouraged to refer to the Children's Workbook as it can serve as a reminder and review of cognitive and behavioral strategies that were successful during treatment and what to do when new OCBs arise, or old OCBs re-emerge.

Pharmacological Treatment

The child's medical practitioner may explore pharmacological treatment with Fb-CBT (or other psychosocial treatments). Each child's full range of diagnoses and medical conditions need to be considered to determine if an additive treatment is needed. Professionals involved with the child should collaborate in a multidisciplinary team to make coordinated and comprehensive treatment decisions.

Our Research That Established Efficacy of Fb-CBT

This research has been primarily guided by an acknowledged clinical need and a large gap in the research literature. Our research goals were two-fold: (a) to gain an understanding of these complex behavioral topographies and create an evidence-based treatment program to reduce OCBs and increase the quality of life for children and their families, and (b) to develop an efficacious treatment and best-practice manuals (including a Children's Workbook) that could be disseminated to practitioners to assist with these prevalent behaviors. Our ultimate goal was to create manuals that could be used *as is* with the confidence that they work.

Since 2007, our OCB research lab's line of study has been carefully guided by an integrated system of science-based practice proposed by Hayes et al. (1999) with a gradual building of research from observational case study work to single-case experimental designs to a preliminary RCT of our group treatment package, culminating in a full RCT of group-based treatment (Vause, Jaksic et al., 2020).

Notably, this is the first RCT to evaluate a manualized treatment package (with individualized training) to reduce OCBs in autism. The RCT included 37 children and youth (7–13 years of age) who were randomly assigned to one of two groups: the Experimental group, meaning they received our nine-week manualized treatment, or the Treatment

As Usual group, meaning they could continue receiving any treatment they were already engaging in but did not access Fb-CBT. Fb-CBT was offered to the Treatment As Usual group after the experimental group completed the trial.

Our two primary standardized measures – Children's Yale-Brown Obsessive Compulsive Scale (CY-BOCS; Goodman et al., 1986) and Repetitive Behavior Scale – Revised (RBS-R; Bodfish et al., 1999) – both showed statistically significant differences at post-test between the Experimental and Treatment As Usual groups with large corrected effect sizes (Hedge's g = 1.00 and 1.15). Our secondary measures (COIS-RP and RBS 100) also showed medium to large corrected effect sizes (Hedge's g = 0.77 and 1.03, respectively). In other words, our Fb-CBT treatment showed efficacy in decreasing targeted OCBs, and maintenance was demonstrated at six-month and five- to seven-year follow-up.

The following graph depicts the changes in OCBs between the Experimental and Treatment As Usual groups across our four measures: Repetitive Behavior Scale – Revised (RBS-R; Sameness, Compulsive, and Ritualistic subscales; Bodfish et al., 1999), Children's Yale-Brown

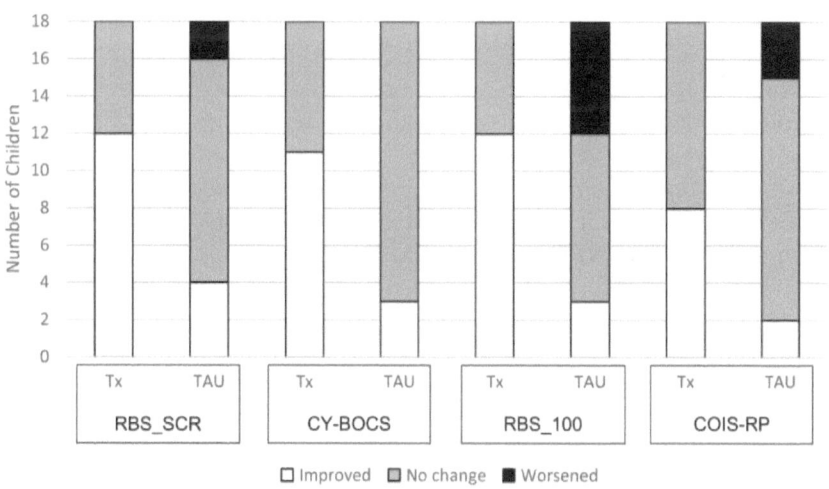

Figure 1.15 Differences between Treatment (Tx) and Treatment As Usual (TAU) scores across four OCB measures (Repetitive Behavior Scale – Revised [RBS_SCR]; Children's Yale-Brown Obsessive Compulsive Scale [CY-BOCS]; Repetitive Behavior Scale – Revised 1–100 [RBS-R_100]; Child Obsessive-Compulsive Impact Scale – Revised Caregiver [COIS-RP]).

Obsessive Compulsive Scale (CY-BOCS; Goodman et al., 1986), Repetitive Behavior Scale – Revised (RBS-R 100; Bodfish et al., 1999), and the Child Obsessive-Compulsive Impact Scale – Revised Caregiver (COIS-RP; Piacentini, Peris et al., 2007). It is noteworthy that there was no worsening of any behavior (black bars) in the experimental group at post-testing. Further, improvements were much more likely for each measure (white bars) in the Experimental group compared to the Treatment As Usual group.

Caregiver Report Data

A Likert scale ranging from 1 (desired post-treatment levels of OCBs) to 3 (partial improvement from pre-treatment levels) to 5 (pre-treatment levels of OCBs) was used by caregivers to give daily ratings of individual OCBs during baseline, treatment, and at follow-up (one and six months). A score of 1 or 2 was recorded as a positive treatment response. Caregivers of children in the Fb-CBT group rated 100 treated behaviors with a mean of 6.25 behaviors per child. Across 16 participants in Fb-CBT, 66% of behaviors that underwent Phase 2 (individualized treatment) showed a decrease to 1 or 2, indicating that the caregivers observed a positive treatment response.

Consumer Satisfaction

Fourteen of the 16 caregivers who were involved in experimental group reported that they were satisfied with the therapy's effectiveness (M = 5.67 [SD = 1.76] on a 7-point Likert scale with a score of 1 being *not at all satisfied* and 7 being *very satisfied* (Vause, Jaksic et al., 2020).

This definitive RCT (Vause, Jaksic et al., 2020) was published in the *Journal of Autism and Developmental Disorders*.

Follow-Up Data Collected Five to Seven Years Later

Using a mixed method design, a follow-up study (Bishop et al., 2024) evaluated the maintenance effects of Fb-CBT on the reduction of OCBs in autistic children five to seven years post-treatment (mean age = 16.9 years). Of the 37 participants who received Fb-CBT in the RCT, 13 consented to participate in this follow-up study. Random effect covariance estimates demonstrated that results were maintained five to seven years later (0.26, SE = 0.25, t[3812] = 1.06, p = 0.29). Caregivers also filled out the Likert scale from the RCT that ranged from 1 (desired post-treatment levels of OCBs) to 3 (partial improvement from pre-treatment levels) to 5 (pre-treatment levels of OCBs) for OCBs worked on during the original treatment. Data was collected daily for one week. Overall, caregiver report data showed that results were maintained from post-treatment to five- to seven-year follow-up.

Conclusion

It is important to target reduction in interfering OCBs, but equally, if not more important, to ensure improvement in quality of life at post-treatment and years later. This chapter provides an overview of OCB complexity in autism, a detailed explanation of our blended Fb-CBT, treatment adaptations, and an explanation of the general layout of this manual. For more information on Fb-CBT, please see our peer-reviewed journal entry (Vause, Neil & Feldman, 2020) edited by Dr. Fred Volkmar, Yale School of Medicine in the Encyclopedia of Autism Spectrum Disorders, to be continually updated and used as a resource for clinicians and researchers.

References

American Psychiatric Association. (2022). *Diagnostic and statistical manual of mental disorders* (5th ed., text rev.). https://doi.org/10.1176/appi.books.9780890425787

Anderson, B. M., Kozluk, A., Chanel, M., Macdonald, M. A., Friedel, J. E., & Cox, A. D. (2023). Exploring characteristics of interventionist training associated with improved learner outcomes: A meta-analysis. *Journal of Behavioral Education, 0123456789*. https://doi.org/10.1007/s10864-022-09504-2

Anderson, B. M., Vause, T., Tarulli, D., Frijters, J. C., & Feldman, M. (Accepted). Best practices and clinical recommendations for adapted group cognitive behaviour therapy to treat anxiety and obsessive compulsive behaviours in children with autism spectrum disorder. *Journal on Developmental Disabilities*.

Bishop, C., Guertin, E., Anderson, B. M., Vause, T., Frijters, J. C., Neil, N., & Feldman, M. (2024, May). Factors affecting long-term outcomes of Functional Behavior-based CBT in treating obsessive-compulsive behaviors in autistic children. In M. Fryling (Discussant) & N. Neil (Chair), *Research gaps and ethical considerations in literature on obsessive-compulsive behavior in autism.* [Symposium]. Association for Behavior Analysis International Annual Conference, Philadelphia, PA.

Bodfish, J. W., Symons, F. J., & Lewis, M. H. (1999). *The Repetitive Behavior Scale: Test manual.* Western Carolina Center Research Reports.

Bodfish, J. W., Symons, F. J., Parker, D. E., & Lewis, M. H. (2000). Varieties of repetitive behavior in autism. *Journal of Autism and Developmental Disabilities, 30*, 237–243.

Boyd, B. A., McDonough, S. G., & Bodfish, J. W. (2012). Evidence-based behavioral interventions for repetitive behaviors in autism. *Journal of Autism and Developmental Disorders, 42*(6), 1236–1248. https://doi.org/10.1007/s10803-011-1284-z

Carr, E. G., & Durand, V. M. (1985). Reducing behavior problems through functional communication training. *Journal of Applied Behavior Analysis, 18*(2), 111–126. https://doi.org/10.1901/jaba.1985.18-111

Chok, J. T., & Harper, J. M. (2016). Heart rate assessment and use of a multiple schedule treatment for an individual with obsessive compulsive-like behavior. *Journal of Developmental and Physical Disabilities, 28*(6), 821–834. https://doi.org/10.1007/s10882-016-9511-3

Franklin, M. E., Freeman, J. B., & March, J. S. (2019). *Treating OCD in children and adolescents: A cognitive-behavioral approach*. Guilford Press.

Goodman, W. K., Price, L. H., Rasmussen, S. A., Riddle, M. A., & Rapoport, J. L. (1986). *Children's yale-brown obsessive compulsive scale (CY-BOCS)*. National Institute of Mental Health.

Guertin, E. L., Vause, T., Thomson, K. M., Frijters, J. C., & Feldman, M. A. (2022). Obsessive–compulsive behaviors in autism spectrum disorder: Behavior analytic conceptual frameworks. *Behavior Analysis: Research and Practice*, Advance online publication. https://doi.org/10.1037/bar0000236

Hanley, G. P., Jin, C. S., Vanselow, N. R., & Hanratty, L. A. (2014). Producing meaningful improvements in problem behavior of children with autism via synthesized analyses and treatments. *Journal of Applied Behavior Analysis, 47*(1), 16–36. https://doi.org/10.1002/jaba.106

Harrop, C., Amsbary, J., Towner-Wright, S., Reichow, B., & Boyd, B. A. (2019). That's what I like: The use of circumscribed interests within interventions for individuals with autism spectrum disorder: A systematic review. *Research in Autism Spectrum Disorders, 57*, 63–86. https://doi.org/10.1016/j.rasd.2018.09.008

Hayes, S. C., Strosahl, K. D., & Wilson, K. G. (1999). *Acceptance and commitment therapy: An experiential approach to behavior change*. Guilford Press.

Ishikawa, S. I., Okajima, I., Matsuoka, H., & Sakano, Y. (2007). Cognitive behavioural therapy for anxiety disorders in children and adolescents: A meta-analysis. *Child and Adolescent Mental Health, 12*(4), 164–172. https://doi.org/10.1111/j.1475-3588.2006.00433.x

Jaksic, H., Vause, T., Frijters, J. C., & Feldman, M. (2018). A comparison of a novel application of hierarchical linear modeling and nonparametric analysis for single-subject designs. *Behavior Analysis: Research and Practice, 18*(2), 203–218. https://doi.org/10.1037/bar0000091

Kinnaird, E., Stewart, C., & Tchanturia, K. (2019). Investigating alexithymia in autism: A systematic review and meta-analysis. *European Psychiatry, 55*, 80–89. https://doi.org/10.1016/j.eurpsy.2018.09.004

Klin, A., Saulnier, C. A., Sparrow, S. S., Cicchetti, D. V., Volkmar, F. R., & Lord, C. (2007). Social and communication abilities and disabilities in higher functioning individuals with autism spectrum disorders: The Vineland and the ADOS. *Journal of Autism and Developmental Disorders, 37*(4), 748–759. https://doi.org/10.1007/s10803-006-0229-4

Lane, K. L., Royer, D. J., Messenger, M. L., Common, E. A., Ennis, R. P., & Swogger, E. D. (2015). Empowering teachers with low-intensity strategies to support academic engagement: Implementation and effects of instructional choice for elementary students in inclusive settings. *Education & Treatment of Children, 38*(4), 473–504. https://doi.org/10.1353/etc.2015.001

March, J. S., & Mulle, K. (1998). *OCD in children and adolescents: A cognitive-behavioral treatment manual*. Guilford Press.

Martin, G., & Pear, J. J. (2024). *Behavior modification: What is it and how to do it* (12th ed.). Routledge.

Mathur, S. K., Renz, E., & Tarbox, J. (2024). Affirming neurodiversity within applied behavior analysis. *Behavior Analysis in Practice, 17*, 471–485. https://doi.org/10.1007/s40617-024-00907-3

Miltenberger, R. G. (2005). The role of automatic negative reinforcement in clinical problems. *International Journal of Behavioral Consultation and Therapy, 1*(1), 1–11. https://doi.org/10.1037/h0100729

Minshawi, N. F., Hurwitz, S., Fodstad, J. C., Biebl, S., Morriss, D. H., & McDougle, C. J. (2014). The association between self-injurious behaviors and autism spectrum disorders. *Psychology Research and Behavior Management, 7,* 125–136. https://doi.org/10.2147/PRBM.S44635

Morris, S., O'Reilly, G., & Nayyar, J. (2021). Classroom-based peer interventions targeting autism ignorance, prejudice and/or discrimination: A systematic PRISMA review. *International Journal of Inclusive Education, 27*(13), 1389–1433. https://doi.org/10.1080/13603116.2021.1900421

National Autism Center. (2015). *National standards project, Phase 2*. May Institute. https://nationalautismcenter.org/national-standards/phase-2-2015/

Parsons, M. B., Rollyson, J. H., & Reid, D. H. (2012). Evidence-based staff training: A guide for practitioners. *Behavior Analysis in Practice, 5*(2), 2–11. https://doi.org/10.1007/BF03391819

Piacentini, J., Langley, A., & Roblek, T. (2007). *Overcoming childhood OCD: A cognitive behavioral treatment program*. Oxford University Press.

Piacentini, J., Peris, T. S., Bergman, R. L., Chang, S., & Jaffer, M. (2007). Brief report: Functional impairment in childhood OCD: Development and psychometrics properties of the Child Obsessive-Compulsive Impact Scale-Revised (COIS-R). *Journal of Clinical Child and Adolescent Psychology, 36*(4), 645–653. https://10.1080/15374410701662790

Reaven, J., Blakeley-Smith, A., Culhane-Shelburne, K., & Hepburn, S. (2012). Group cognitive behavior therapy for children with high-functioning autism spectrum disorders and anxiety: A randomized trial. *Journal of Child Psychology and Psychiatry, and Allied Disciplines, 53*(4), 410–419. https://doi.org/10.1111/j.1469-7610.2011.02486.x

Reaven, J., & Hepburn, S. (2003). Cognitive-behavioral treatment of obsessive-compulsive disorder in a child with Asperger syndrome: A case report. *Autism, 7*(2), 145–164. https://doi.org/10.1177/1362361303007002003

Reutebuch, C. K., El Zein, F., & Roberts, G. J. (2015). A systematic review of the effects on choice on academic outcomes for students with autism spectrum disorder. *Research in Autism Spectrum Disorders, 20,* 1–16. https://doi.org/10.1016/j.rasd.2015.08.002

Sarokoff, R. A., & Sturmey, P. (2008). The effects of instructions, rehearsal, modeling, and feedback on acquisition and generalization of staff use of discrete trial teaching and student correct responses. *Research in Autism Spectrum Disorders, 2*(1), 125–136. https://doi.org/10.1016/j.rasd.2007.04.002

Scarpa, A., White, S. W., & Attwood, T. (2016). *CBT for children and adolescents with high-functioning autism spectrum disorders*. Guilford Press.

Schnabel, A., Youssef, G. J., Hallford, D. J., Hartley, E. J., McGillivray, J. A., Stewart, M., Forbes, D., & Austin, D. W. (2020). Psychopathology in caregivers of children with autism spectrum disorder: A systematic review and meta-analysis of prevalence. *Autism: The International Journal of Research and Practice, 24*(1), 26–40. https://doi.org/10.1177/1362361319844636

Schwartz, J. M. (1997). *Brain lock: Free yourself from obsessive-compulsive behavior*. Harper Perennial.

South, M., Ozonoff, S., & McMahon, W. M. (2005). Repetitive behavior profiles in Asperger syndrome and high-functioning autism. *Journal of Autism and Developmental Disorders, 35*(2), 145–158. https://doi.org/10.1007/s10803-004-1992-8

Steinbrenner, J. R., Hume, K., Odom, S. L., Morin, K. L., Nowell, S. W., Tomaszewski, B., Szendrey, S., Mcintyre, N. S., Yucesoy-Ozkan, S., & Savage, M. N. (2020). *Evidence-based practices for children, youth, and young adults with autism*. The National Clearinghouse on Autism Evidence and Practice Review Team.

Stone, W. S., & Chen, G. (2016). Comorbidity of autism spectrum and obsessive-compulsive disorders. *North American Journal of Medicine and Science, 8*(3), 109–112. https://doi.org/10.7156/najms. 2015.0803109

Taylor, S., & Jang, K. L. (2011). Biopsychosocial etiology of obsessions and compulsions: An integrated behavioral-genetic and cognitive-behavioral analysis. *Journal of Abnormal Psychology, 120*(1), 174–186. https://doi.org/10.1037/a0021403

Toussaint, K. A., Kodak, T., & Vladescu, J. C. (2016). An evaluation of choice on instructional efficacy and individual preferences among children with autism. *Journal of Applied Behavior Analysis, 49*(1), 170–175. https://doi.org/10.1002/jaba.263

Twomey, M. (2020). Can you hear me? Accessing the voice of the child with Autism and their parent. *Educação, 43*(1), 35477. https://doi.org/10.15448/1981-2582.2020.1.35477

Unguru, Y. (2011). Pediatric decision-making: Informed consent, parental permission, and child assent. *Clinical Ethics in Pediatrics: A Case-Based Textbook,* 1–6. https://doi.org/10.1017/CBO9780511740336.002

Vause, T., Hoekstra, S., & Feldman, M. (2014). Evaluation of individual function-based cognitive-behavioural therapy for obsessive compulsive behaviour in children with autism spectrum disorder. *Journal on Developmental Disabilities, 20*(3), 30–41.

Vause, T., Jaksic, H., Neil, N., Frijters, J. C., Jackiewicz, G., & Feldman, M. (2020). Functional behavior-based cognitive-behavioral therapy for obsessive compulsive behavior in children with autism spectrum disorder: A randomized controlled trial. *Journal of Autism and Developmental Disorders, 50*(7), 2375–2388. https://doi.org/10.1007/s10803-018-3772-x

Vause, T., Neil, N., & Feldman, M. (2020). *Functional behavior-based cognitive-behavioral therapy for obsessive-compulsive behavior in children with ASD*. In F. R. Volkmar (Ed.), *Encyclopedia of Autism spectrum disorders*. Springer. https://doi.org/10.1007/978-1-4614-6435-8_102481-1

Vause, T., Neil, N., Jaksic, H., Jackiewicz, G., & Feldman, M. (2017). Preliminary randomized trial of function-based cognitive-behavioral therapy to treat obsessive compulsive behavior in children with autism spectrum disorder. *Focus on Autism and Other Developmental Disabilities, 32*(3), 218–228. https://doi.org/10.1177/1088357615588517

Vella, L., Ring, H. A., Aitken, M. R., Watson, P. C., Presland, A., & Clare, I. C. (2018). Understanding self-reported difficulties in decision-making by people with autism spectrum disorders. *Autism, 22*(5), 549–559. https://doi.org/10.1177/136236131668798

Whitbourne, S. K. (2023). *Abnormal psychology: Clinical perspectives on psychological disorders* (10th ed.). McGraw Hill Education.

Wood, J., Drahota, A., Sze, K., Har, K., Chiv, A., & Langer, D. (2009). Cognitive behavioral therapy for anxiety in children with autism spectrum disorders: A randomized, controlled trial. *Journal of Child Psychology and Psychiatry, 50*(3), 224–234. https://doi.org/10.1111/j.1469-7610.2008.01948.x

Wood, R. (2023). Autism, intense interests and support in school: From wasted efforts to shared understandings. In J. Martin, M. Bowl, & G. Banks (Eds.), *Mapping the field: 75 years of educational review* (pp. 21–23). Routledge.

Appendix A

Adaptations to Support Autistic Children

Table 1.2 Adaptations to Support Autistic Children

Fb-CBT Adaptation	Description
Caregiver Involvement	Intensive caregiver involvement in assessment and treatment sessions is highly recommended to provide encouragement and coaching to generalize strategies from the clinic to home and other environments.
Structure and Predictability	Fb-CBT encourages a consistent weekly routine with a visual schedule and consistent opening and closing activities.
Use of Visuals	Visuals are embedded into the Children's Workbook to accommodate varying cognitive, speech, and learning profiles. They assist with offering various ways to communicate (e.g., writing, coloring), emotion recognition, explaining concepts, and providing reinforcement (e.g., checkmarks, use of a token board). It allows for flexibility to promote individualized treatment.
Simplifying Language and Using Concrete Language When Needed	Use short, simple sentences when communicating. Use concrete examples to explain concepts and constructs. Consider a combination of forced-choice questions and open-ended questions, as appropriate for the child.
Incorporation of Interests and Preoccupations	Modify worksheets or visuals to include the child's preoccupations and interests. Frame scenarios or examples using preferred characters or elements from the child's favorite movies, books, or games.
Emotion Recognition Training	Use emotion cards (e.g., faces depicting emotions) and visuals in Fb-CBT workbook to help identify emotions and physiological sensations. Engage in role-playing exercises where the child practices identifying emotions and responding appropriately. Create opportunities and provide positive feedback and reinforcement when the individual identifies emotions.

(Continued)

Table 1.2 (Continued)

Fb-CBT Adaptation	Description
Incorporating Child Voice	Give each child the right to express themselves in their preferred modality (e.g., using their voice, a communication device, gestures, or facial expressions). Ongoing assent/consent should occur throughout treatment.
Personalized Coping Techniques	Personalized coping techniques can help provide calming/soothing/anxiety reduction properties and/or offer a "replacement" for the compulsion. Children may use active coping techniques (e.g., exercising or muscle relaxation) and/or passive strategies (e.g., reading a book).
Functional Communication Training	After identifying perceived functions (see Chapter 3), functional replacement behaviors can be put in place. Formalized programming such as functional communication training can be used to teach children how to access what they want (e.g., how to initiate a conversation to access social attention).
Protracted Self-Talk and Cognitive Restructuring	You may address "probability" on a basic level and relate this to prosocial behavior. You may also examine prosocial behaviors that people in the child's life engage in (e.g., eating healthy, exercising, taking safety precautions). For personal responsibility, help the child to see that there are many reasons why events happen and that they are largely out of the child's control. Self-talk can be derived on its own or from ideas/reframing of thoughts during cognitive restructuring.
Gradual Exposure and Breaking OCBs into Multiple Steps as Needed.	Gradually expose the child in E/RP and allow them an active role in determining the exposure steps. Anxiety exposure/distress will occur in small doses to prevent overwhelming them (and decreasing child and caregiver motivation). Gradual exposure allows for small successes with *some* anxiety leading in many cases to the elimination of OCBs.
Token Systems and Thinning Delivery of Reinforcement	Provide immediate feedback when the child is successful with session activities. Encourage caregivers to use verbal praise, high-fives, or a preferred item/activity as a reward for using coping techniques and practicing exposures. Use a token system for each session and encourage use at home. As children gain control over OCBs, the delivery of reinforcement should be thinned or faded to more naturalistic consequences.

Appendix B

Reinforcer Checklist

Learner's Name: _____   Date: _____

Check off the items/activities the learner enjoys. Add in any items/activities not on list

Edibles
___ Candy
___ Chocolate
___ Chips
___ Crackers
___ Cereal
___ Fruit
___ Vegetables
___ Cheese
___ Meat
___ Ice cream
___ Popsicle
___ Pudding
___ Juice
___ Pop/soda
___ Other: _____
___ Other: _____
___ Other: _____

Tangibles
___ Bubbles
___ Spin toys
___ Bean bags
___ Balls
___ Puzzles
___ Balloons
___ Play dough
___ Stickers
___Stamps
___ Instruments
___ Blocks
___ Sensory bin
___ Light up toy
___ Remote controlled car
___ Car ramp
___ Other: _____
___ Other: _____
___ Other: _____

Games/Sports
___ Baseball
___ Soccer
___ Basketball
___ Bicycle
___ Board game
___ Card game
___ Tag
___ Playground
___ Follow the leader
___ Tag
___ Bean bag toss
___ Other: _____
___ Other: _____
___ Other: _____

Electronics
___ Watch a movie
___ Computer
___ Videogame
___ Phone
___ Tablet
___ Calculator
___ Watch
___ Smart Board
___ Other: _____
___ Other: _____
___ Other: _____

Events
___ Line leader
___ Peer tutor
___ Break from the room
___ Instructor's helper
___ Free time
___ Other: _____
___ Other: _____
___ Other: _____

Social
___ Singing
___ Hug
___ Praise
___ High five
___ Tickles
___ Read together
___ Back scratch
___ Handshake
___ Whistling
___ Silly faces
___ Telling jokes
___ Making funny voices
___ Playing pretend
___ Other: _____
___ Other: _____
___ Other: _____

Activities
___ Dancing
___ Drawing
___ Trampoline
___ Go for a walk
___ Rocking/spinning
___ Water play
___ Peek-a-boo
___ Taking pictures
___ Treasure hunt
___ Wagon ride
___ Swinging
___ Relay race
___ Dress up
___ Sandbox
___ Bug collecting
___ Show and tell
___ Other: _____
___ Other: _____
___ Other: _____

Figure 1.16 Reinforcer assessment.

Chapter 2

Clinical Assessment

Introduction

As a core domain of autism, repetitive and restrictive behaviors (RRBs) assume a vast number of topographies (or forms) among autistic children. As discussed in Chapter 1, RRBs in autism can be divided into two broad subtypes of repetitive behavior: lower-order and higher-order RRBs (Bodfish et al., 2000; Mirenda et al., 2010). Research supports higher-order RRBs such as *compulsions* (e.g., ordering and arranging), rituals (e.g., rigid routines, repetitive questioning), and *sameness* behavior (e.g., sitting in the same place) in autism loading on the same factor (Mirenda et al., 2010). Higher-order RRBs show similar topographies to symptoms of obsessive-compulsive disorder (OCD). In other words, many of these repetitive behaviors may serve to mitigate anxiety or may be performed in response to an established rule on the part of the child (APA, 2022). The performance of these behaviors often causes daily interference for the child and their family members, educational and social barriers, and increased caregiver stress (Boyd et al., 2012; Vause, Jaksic et al., 2020).

When these behaviors arise, we first conduct a detailed clinical assessment. During the clinical or diagnostic assessment, a clinician will attempt to differentiate lower-order RRBs from higher-order RRBs. Then, if applicable and desired by the child and family, the therapist can design an individualized treatment to address the perceived functions, including anxiety reduction and other contributing variables (e.g., accessing social attention). In this assessment chapter, we offer the following:

- A review of obsessive-compulsive behavior (OCB), potential operant functions, and consideration of individual variables;
- Two clinical cases with varying assessment information offered from the child or youth regarding the OCB;
- General and probe-specific assessment considerations;

DOI: 10.4324/9781003410126-2

- A clinical walk through for assessing OCBs based on our randomized controlled trial (RCT); and
- Considerations for diagnosis (if in one's scope of practice) and the complex nature of assessing behaviors with covert components in autistic individuals.

Worksheets are then provided with recommendations of a step-by-step process for narrowing down what OCBs to treat, given the level of interference and other factors. A caregiver data sheet for OCBs is also provided.

Assessing Obsessive-Compulsive Behavior With a Comprehensive Clinical Assessment

As described in Chapter 1, we use the term obsessive-compulsive behaviors, or OCBs, to refer to higher-order RRBs that may serve to reduce anxiety but also may be maintained by other functional variables (e.g., access to social attention, sensory stimulation, removing a nonpreferred task or activity, or accessing a preferred stimulus). Recall one of our key diagrams in Chapter 1 to review the overlapping nature and functions of OCBs.

When assessing and programming for OCBs, challenges may arise, such as varying degrees of self-awareness and difficulty in describing thoughts, emotions, feelings, and bodily sensations (e.g., Franklin et al., 2019; March & Mulle, 1998). These challenges begin as early as the assessment stage. It is our experience that many children become

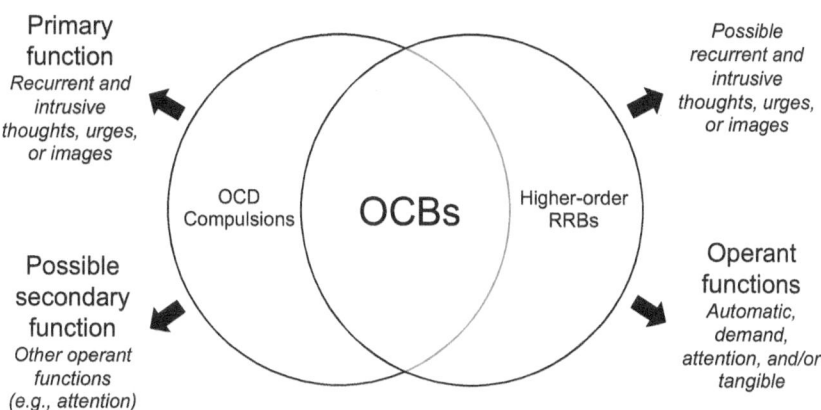

Figure 2.1 Operant function(s) and the overlapping nature of OCBs.

increasingly fluent in these socio-emotional skills related to OCBs as we continue to break them down into smaller components over sessions and engage in practical exercises throughout treatment.

We view the assessment process as a learning-to-learn assessment and an opportunity to gather information about the child and their unique characteristics. Through interacting with a child (and their caregivers), we can (a) begin to familiarize a child with what OCBs are; (b) understand if their challenges fit in the realm of OCBs and their degree of interference; and (c) begin the process of formulating a clinical impression of social-communicative, developmental, and cognitive strengths and challenges that need to be considered throughout the assessment and treatment process. For example, we can gather valuable information on thought processes (e.g., degree of introspection, perspective-taking skills, social-communicative challenges such as engaging in back-and-forth conversational skills, and general processing speed).

Various methods are used to identify perceived operant functions, including standardized clinical assessments and behavioral observation, during clinical assessment. Conducting behavioral observations or having a child self-monitor their OCBs occurs throughout treatment, but we can begin examining maintaining variables for OCBs at this stage. This may be accomplished in several ways, depending on the nature of the behaviors. For example, the therapist may be able to directly observe a behavior, such as repetitive questioning during the assessment, or the child may self-monitor a given behavior at the clinic or at home. It is also possible that they may not present with the prerequisite skills to self-monitor. An in-depth discussion of behavioral observation is provided in Chapter 3, with a guide on conducting a functional behavioral assessment.

When formulating clinical impressions, the therapist must listen carefully to how the youth describes their compulsions and obsessions and the words they use and repeat. The therapist must also consider when further probing is needed, and the general environmental context. As a clinical assessor, you may ask yourself the following questions to maximize descriptive data. First, can the client clearly describe the compulsion (and obsession if present)? Is further probing needed, and what type may be helpful? Might different communication modalities (e.g., drawing) support them? Through careful note-taking and behavioral observation, the therapist can gather a plethora of information on the clinical presentation of the client, as well as strengths and potential challenges. If intrusive thoughts (see Figure 2.1) are present, what kinds of connections can the child draw between the compulsion and obsession? In

Chapter 1 (see Two Types of OCB), we discussed two flavors of OCD where obsessions may be related to a "not just right" feeling that drives the performance of the compulsion or worries about something bad happening to oneself or others (March and Mulle, 1998).

In exploring obsessions and compulsions, we are primarily attempting to target the anxiety piece of the puzzle (e.g., thoughts, feelings, physiological responses). What about an initial consideration of other contributing variables? For compulsions, does the child talk about or allude to accessing variables such as caregiver attention or avoiding an unwanted task (like checking their bag in replacement of helping with family tasks to get ready for an outing)? Do they talk about lining materials up and admiring the lineup of their preferred items in a particular order (e.g., stuffed animals)? Can you observe these behaviors in session through conversation with the child and caregivers and/or with stimuli brought into the clinic room? Additional questioning and behavioral observation may be necessary with autistic children to begin the process of identifying potential contributing variables that may assist with the comprehensive functional behavioral assessment (described in Chapter 3), clinical programming, and possible "rule-outs" of behaviors based on function and psychiatric disorders or other presenting challenges.

Table 2.1 presents selected examples of compulsive behavior frequently encountered in our work with children and youth. For each behavior, we consider anxiety as well as other operant functions. The first bullet point offers questions about anxiety. The latter bullet points may assist a clinician in exploring other potential variables.

Beginning to explore behaviors maintained by anxiety and delving into other perceived functions beyond anxiety (i.e., social attention, access to tangible, escape/avoidance, sensory stimulation) may aid a therapist in starting to rule out functions or determine if there are multiple functions present. For example, in the case of sitting in the same seat, the child may say, "I don't feel right" if they do not engage in this behavior, but it may also give them a good view of the caregivers' body and face such that it is easier to view the caregiver and engage in a conversation. This may lead a therapist to note and continue to assess both variables (anxiety reduction and social attention from the caregiver) as contributing factors when conducting an in-depth functional behavior assessment (see Chapter 3).

Referring to Table 2.1, there is often a need to carefully analyze statements when determining underlying functions (e.g., rules that a child states when playing a game and whether this is related to controlling the outcome of the game). Consideration of other functions and the context

Table 2.1 Examples of OCBs and Consideration of Function

Behavior	Therapist Considerations/Thoughts Regarding Function(s)
Insistence on being first into public areas with caregivers and siblings	• Anxiety reduction function – Is an observable or reported tension/anxiety for the child created if this regimented order is not present during most occurrences? How is this expressed (e.g., vocally or selected physiological responses)? • Tangible function – The therapist may ask questions related to variables such as being the first person to access tangibles (e.g., ordering food in a restaurant first or accessing apparatus in a playground). Does this appear more when preferred stimuli are present?
Insistence on playing a game in a certain way and others responding in a manner dictated by the child	• Anxiety reduction function – Is this related to a "not just right" obsession/tension? Does the child insist that rules listed in a manual be explicitly followed? • Tangible function – Does the child insist on following selective rules to help them win? • Analyzing the child's statements and patterns of responding, as well as the connection between rules and controlling access to game outcomes, may help the therapist draw hypotheses/conclusions.
Insistence on taking the same route to a destination	• Anxiety reduction function – Is this related to a "not just right" obsession/tension if the same route is not taken on every occasion? • Tangible function – Does the route the child insists on following pass by their favorite fast-food restaurant? If the child has a favorite location en route but has frequent access to it (e.g., McDonald's), does the child's expressed need to go the same route decrease?
Insistence on wearing certain pieces of clothing	• Anxiety reduction function – Is this related to a "not just right" feeling when wearing clothes that are not a certain color or texture daily? • Sensory function – Does the child describe clothes as cozy and comfortable?
Repetitive checking of backpack	• Anxiety reduction function – Is this related to anxiety around ensuring items are in certain places or "just right"? • Tangible function – Does the child check that the backpack has all the items they may need to access or play with? • Escape function – Does the child escape from doing a nonpreferred activity or chore by repeatedly checking their backpack?
Sitting in the same seat	• Anxiety reduction function – Is this related to a "not just right" obsession/tension if not sitting in a certain seat? • Tangible function – Does the child enjoy the view from the preferred seat or can the child access favorable items like USB ports/car play or other devices? • Attention function – Does the seat give the child a better view of the front driver (e.g., caregiver) to engage in conversation with them?

(Continued)

Table 2.1 (Continued)

Behavior	Therapist Considerations/Thoughts Regarding Function(s)
Repetitive questioning	• Anxiety reduction function – Does the child appear anxious if not able to engage in repeating the same question multiple times? Does the child ask the caregiver to repeat back a response in a regimented manner and provide reassurance? • Tangible function – Is the child more likely to get what they are asking for if they repeatedly ask their caregivers for it? • Attention function – Does the child smile before, during, or after engaging in the response? • Attention function – Does the child receive more and immediate caregiver attention when they repeat questions than when they do not?

in which the behavior occurs allows the therapist to examine multiple layers and attempt to unpack, at times, some very complex chains of behavior. This may mean going above and beyond a traditional assessment of OCB (e.g., Children's Yale-Brown Obsessive Compulsive Scale [CY-BOCS; Goodman et al., 1986] or other standardized instruments) but could provide more in-depth knowledge to assist with ruling out behaviors and further assessment to develop an individualized treatment program for an OCB. This chapter also describes other "rule-outs" of disorders and references to the *Diagnostic and Statistical Manual of Mental Disorders, Fifth Edition, Text Revision* (DSM-5-TR; APA, 2022) that may share similar features such as anxiety disorders, skin picking, trichotillomania, and Tourette's Syndrome. In these cases, referral or consultation with a trained professional in ruling out other diagnoses is necessary.

We now present two unique case presentations of children and youth seen in our clinic, as well as therapist considerations and reflections regarding the information offered by these clients and the behaviors observed.

Clinical Case Conceptualization 1: 14-Year-Old Jess, Presence of Compulsions With Associated Obsessions

At intake, the initial responses of 14-year-old Jess regarding his description of compulsions and related obsessions provided preliminary insight into possible contributing variables (see Figure 2.1). Jess was referred for treatment because of his fear of his food not digesting and needing to engage in compulsions to alleviate anxiety. At first, he was hesitant to vocally contribute. With encouragement and assistance from his father to describe his OCBs, he offered partial explanations of his fears related to his food not digesting and vocalized his intense fear of food particles "getting stuck." Further probing and assistance from his father aided in adding supplemental information regarding his obsessional fears and related compulsions (e.g., reassurance in the form of repetitive questioning that he was not going to choke). His father helped with forming clear connections between obsessions and compulsions that Jess believed he needed to perform. A more in-depth description was gathered by asking for more information and relying on his father's assistance. Jess would frequently ask, "Dad, is that right?"

In Jess's case, the father helped to add information to the youth's description, and he would often confirm or disconfirm the information (which is an example of working together to maximize the depth and breadth of information). The youth was also able to describe clear connections between antecedents (e.g., eating hard foods), obsessions (e.g., fear of choking or food particles getting stuck in his stomach), and related compulsions (reassurance through repetitive question-asking of his father and others, and/or patting his stomach to "make the food go down"). Referring to our conceptual framework in Figure 2.1, the primary variable of anxiety reduction (negative reinforcement) was apparent. However, additional contributing variables were directly observed by the therapist such as frequently accessing his father's attention with questions, comments, and nonvocal behavior (e.g., eye contact and smiling) related to this persistent OCB. Jess appeared anxious (e.g., blinking, patting stomach) when describing OCBs, but he also smiled at his father when discussing the compulsions. He had developed elaborate conversational scripts around the OCB concerning digestion and types of food to eat.

Box 2.1   Quote From Martin and Pear (2024)
Regarding Attention as an Operant Function

"Indicators that the behavior is maintained by attention include (a) whether attention reliably follows the behavior; (b) whether the individual looks at or approaches a caregiver just before engaging in the behavior; and (c) whether the individual smiles just before engaging in the behavior" (p. 229, 2024).

When further examining Jess' overall conversational repertoire, although conversational questions for this OCB were numerous and fluent, this youth experienced considerable difficulty engaging in conversation related to other topics, including his preferred interests and preoccupations (e.g., sports statistics) and making small talk (e.g., talking about his day). Nonverbal behaviors (e.g., smiling), the caregiver attention Jess received after engaging in OCB-related behavior, and the recognizable challenge of maintaining a conversation led the therapist to hypothesize a second functional variable, which was access to his father's attention by discussing his OCB. This youth would repeatedly ask for information about digestion and pose questions such as: *"Will my food digest? Why is my stomach making funny noises? Is this a hard food? Am I going to be OK?"*

Clinical Case Conceptualization 2: 10-Year-Old Alice, Presence of Compulsions With No Obsessions Vocalized

Alice was referred for treatment for her repetitive ordering, arranging, and needing to have items "just so." Her parents acknowledged that there was a history of OCD and anxiety disorders in both the immediate and extended families. During the assessment, it was difficult for Alice to discuss her compulsions (and possible related obsessions). When the triggering stimuli were present (e.g., stuffed animals), Alice was more likely to describe compulsions (and the chain of behaviors she engaged in) and acknowledge their presence. There were varying types of OCBs that were readily observed with a large class of OCBs involving "ordering and arranging." This school-age child was regularly observed to (a) arrange multiple items (e.g., stuffed animals) in her bedroom and classroom at school where persons could not touch the items; (b) need her personal items such as her water bottle to remain in the same location; (c) engage in complex regimented routines (e.g., a seven-step morning routine that needed to occur in the same order each time); and (d) immediately interrupt any disruption to her compulsions by others (including her parents) with a display of visible agitation. Agitation involved vocal statements (e.g., fussing/whining, insisting the person stop moving objects she arranged) and nonvocal behaviors (pulling and fluffing her hair, facial redness) until the materials were returned to their original location. Alice engaged in OCBs for more than one hour per day, which impeded her participation in, and enjoyment of, social and individual activities that she preferred. Reflecting on the two flavors of OCD (something bad happening and "not just right" behavior), it appeared that if things were "not just right," Alice needed to arrange and order objects with anxiety relief as a potentially contributing variable (see Figure 2.1).

During the ongoing assessment, the clinician asked the school staff (who had established good rapport with this child) to ask about the thoughts immediately before and during the compulsion. Alice would often get upset and, a few times, verbalized, "I just need to, OK?" which is a common response for many children. Parents attempted to discuss the compulsion with Alice to determine the triggering obsession, but she reported no obsessions. Interestingly, this child was verbally fluent, could discuss preferred and nonpreferred topics in depth, and put forth detailed opinion statements. However, her reduced level of introspection and self-awareness may have impacted her ability to express information concerning her obsessions/thoughts (APA, 2022).

Given the absence of thoughts/obsessions related to compulsions, it was difficult to partial out whether these OCBs were maintained by (a) anxiety/tension and the need to reduce it; (b) access to sensory stimulation, including enjoyment/satisfaction in the way the stimuli looked or appeared in the environment; or (c) a combination of both anxiety reduction and access to internal sensory reinforcement. Given that these behaviors likely contained a covert component (anxiety) but the vocalization of the obsession was not present, it was challenging to determine likely functions. Nonetheless, it is important to consider the following variables: (a) Alice presented with several OCBs that involved ordering and rearranging; (b) she had a history of OCD and anxiety in her family; (c) she engaged in other OCBs outside of this ordering/arranging stimulus class subset; and (d) these behaviors interfered daily in the lives of herself and others such that they often prevented her from engaging in preferred activities in everyday life.

In carefully considering possible functional variables, our functional behavior-based cognitive behavioral therapy (Fb-CBT) was implemented across several settings. We were unsure as to the relative contribution of maintaining variables but observed functional impairment and a considerable impact on the quality of life of Alice and her family members. Using cognitive behavioral therapy (CBT) skills training and gradual exposure with response prevention (see Chapter 1), Alice learned coping mechanisms to use in replacement of agitation, such as taking deep breaths and having conversations with people, how/when she could satisfy her needs (e.g., ordering with activities such as puzzles, arranging some personal belongings that she carried with her, and accessing internal sensory stimulation with pop-up/sensory toys). Although she may have enjoyed the internal sensations of her original OCBs regarding ordering and arranging, she also expressed enjoyment in her increased interaction with family members and peers, having more regular access to her preferred items (beyond those involved in her OCBs), and not feeling "stressed" (a common word she used) in her everyday routines.

Summary of the Clinical Cases

We have now described two clinical cases with children and youth with very different clinical presentations. In the case of repetitive questioning, with the assistance of his father, Jess was able to articulate his compulsions and related obsessions clearly. However, with Alice, the compulsions (arranging various personal items, such as stuffed animals) were usually observable, and she could describe the behavior chain, but she did not share any obsessions. As a clinician, you may be working with more complex presentations, like in the case of Alice, where she could not convey her thoughts. Over many years, we have worked with plenty of children and youth who do not have a thought to accompany a compulsion, have partial thoughts, or have thoughts that emerge during treatment. We often see children where thoughts are present or vocalized for some OCBs and not others. Be mindful that even when a thought is not communicated, similar to Alice and her rearranging, children may show distress (e.g., crying, redness in the face, rapid breathing) when interrupted from engaging in the compulsion.

Continuing to build on the information presented in Chapter 1, this assessment chapter shows the impact of the children's challenges with introspection and awareness of self and others and describing obsessions. These difficulties may be worse if the child is anxious for other reasons during the assessment or has yet to develop rapport with the assessor. In the case of Jess, his father was present to aid in the vocal description of the OCB, add additional information, and confirm/disconfirm information provided by the youth. Even neurotypical children often have difficulty relaying the thoughts/images underlying specific compulsions (APA, 2022; Oar et al., 2017). With standardized assessments and initial behavioral observation, you gather preliminary information from the child. However, you may need to adapt assessment and treatment by breaking down concepts, building rapport, and working on social communicative skills that allow the autistic child to offer additional insight regarding OCBs.

Simply put, OCBs are tricky! Using standardized clinical assessments that list compulsions (and related thoughts/obsessions) like the CY-BOCS to gather information from a behavioral and clinical assessment is important. As a therapist, you must break down the various compulsions (and related obsessions) and take careful notes of relevant examples offered by the child/caregiver. As in the case of Jess, it is often helpful to have a caregiver with the child to assist in describing the OCBs and to offer their observations of the child concerning what they have noticed in different environments. The child or youth may also look to the caregiver for help with clinical descriptions. However, if the child asks the caregiver for assistance, ensure you refer to the child for a "check" of the information (like in the case of Jess) and give ample time to process the information and voice their thoughts. Last, remember that the child or youth may be anxious when encountering a new setting and describing OCBs to an unfamiliar person. Children may enter the assessment room with their faces hidden by clothing (e.g., wearing a hat to cover their face) or position themselves to face the caregiver or at a comfortable distance from the therapist. Rapport building before and throughout the assessment and icebreaker exercises are often helpful in creating a comfortable and relaxing environment. In the case of Alice, working with the identified compulsions and continuing to probe and observe what occurs before the compulsion may or may not give you a glimpse of the obsession. However, it is often worth the attempt.

Strategies and Adaptations for Children With Autism

Tables 2.2 and 2.3 summarize strategies and adaptations for children with autism and related disabilities to consider before and during the assessment process. They include (a) general considerations and (b) adaptations to probe for assessment information and the use of varying communication modalities given the acknowledged difficulty for children in relaying this information (APA, 2022). Many of the general considerations (Table 2.2) and adaptations (Table 2.3) apply to assessment and treatment alike. You may need to be creative in contriving environments that set the stage for the compulsion or engage in role-playing or imaginal exposure. What are some examples of icebreakers or rapport-building exercises that you often use with children? Creative solutions and trying out alternatives are key to gathering more information, determining the level of interference, the child's functional impairment, and how OCBs affect quality of life.

Table 2.2 General Considerations

Considerations	Description
Rapport Building	• Consider conducting a preference assessment. Encourage the caregiver/client to bring preferred items, such as those indicated on the Reinforcement Assessment for Individuals with Severe Disabilities (RAISD; Fisher et al., 1996), to the assessment. • Do an icebreaker exercise or something fun with the child when the child enters the room. For example, the child and caregivers may form a circle, and the clinician stands in the middle. One at a time, the clinician calls out different things the child may enjoy, such as characters, foods, sports, etc. The child and caregiver take turns taking one step forward if they enjoy what the clinician calls out and one step backward if they do not. • Through trial and error or perhaps asking the child/caregiver, explore the child's preferred conversational style and communication with others (e.g., adding in jokes, being asked closed versus open-ended questions, amount/type of eye contact).
Ensure the Child's Voice is Heard	• Prioritize obtaining consent/assent from the child in addition to caregiver consent and reassess regularly. • Provide opportunities for the child to express themselves in their chosen modality. • Recognize the nonverbal ways in which each child's "voice" may be manifested, such as changes in facial expression (e.g., frowning when a particular activity is introduced) or body language (e.g., pointing to what they want). • Provide reassurance and encouragement when the child uses their voice. • Be open-minded and ready to adapt to meet the child's needs, such as shortening a component if the child is distressed.
Use Preferred Modalities of Communication	• During assessment, explore different modalities, such as vocal communication, drawing pictures, sign language, using a computer or other visual aids, using formal communication systems (e.g., P2Go) with vocal communication or alone, and using 3D stimuli to help describe OCBs.
How to Best Access Information from the Child and Caregiver	• If it is the caregiver who is mainly offering information, do frequent checks with the child. This may vary depending on what type of information you are requesting, the age of the child, and other variables.
Offer Breaks and Snacks	• The frequency of breaks may need to be altered throughout the session depending on the type of information asked, the child's level of fatigue, and other individual variables. • Breaks/snacks are recommended when administering assessment instruments as they are often content-heavy.

(Continued)

Table 2.2 (Continued)

Considerations	Description
Break Tasks and Questions down into Smaller Components	• A task that contains multiple steps can be broken down into simpler, individual steps. • If a child is capable but appears to be having trouble identifying their anxious thoughts/feelings during a given assessment, consider administering only one portion and saving the other for a different time. • You may need to use synonyms, break down the wording, or give multiple examples (where needed) if the child does not understand the information (e.g., a compulsion you are describing).
Various Types of Reinforcement	• Explore various types of reinforcement that can be delivered during the assessment process (see preference assessment piece). • How often does reinforcement need to be delivered? Can it be delivered during assessment breaks, or does it need to be interspersed throughout the assessment sections? • Would a token system be helpful? See Positive Reinforcement in Chapter 1.
Addressing Caregiver and Child Anxiety	• Allow the child to position themselves in a way that they are comfortable. You could ask about how much space they need from others, who they would like to sit next to, how they would like to spread out their preferred activities, etc. • Ask the child how they are feeling. Use a visual if this is helpful. Offer coping strategies as needed (e.g., taking deep breaths). It is important to ask the child what they think works for them! • Ask the caregiver(s) about their comfort level. This way, the child does not feel singled out and you can ensure that the caregiver feels as comfortable as possible. You could offer available items (e.g., coffee, tea, water) if allowable in your facility or available in your private practice. • Explain to the caregiver/child that it is typical to feel a sense of discomfort at the beginning and reiterate that OCBs are very common. In our experience, caregivers are sometimes under the assumption that these symptoms are rare. Take the child's lead (e.g., let the child determine when they're ready to approach a fearful situation rather than forcing them to do so). • Remember that even though an autistic child or youth is not making direct eye contact, it doesn't necessarily mean they aren't paying attention.

Table 2.3 Suggestions for Probing for Information Regarding Compulsions and Obsessions

Types of Probes	Description and Examples
General Probes	• You may want to use an assessment that has a **symptom checklist**. Make a note of any modifications you make.
	• A symptom checklist often connects the obsessions with compulsions (e.g., Are you worried about germs getting on you from bugs or people that are ill?) rather than asking separate questions about compulsions and obsessions (Franklin et al., 2019).
	• When needed, you may be required to modify, clarify the wording, or offer synonyms for words if a child or youth does not appear to understand or asks for clarification.
	• If a child has difficulty explaining an obsession, you may probe further by asking questions like "What do you think about right before [compulsion]?"
	• A variety of suggestions are offered by Franklin et al. (2019) concerning different probes you could use. These experts suggest being explicit in your questioning. For example, asking if the compulsion keeps you safe, prevents something bad from happening, or makes you feel safe or better in some way.
Other Probes and Ways to Probe	*Ask the caregiver to observe the child at home and, if feasible, ask about the obsession immediately before, during, or after the compulsion takes place.* A probe could be, "Can you tell me what you thought about right before you [name compulsion]? Depending on the child, a probe may occur before, during or after the compulsion occurs.
	Get an idea of the topography of the OCB with the stimuli present in your clinic. Encourage children/caregivers to bring anxiety provoking/interfering stimuli to the clinic (if they are willing). With the visuals present, have the child walk you through the compulsion with the assistance of a caregiver. Children may also bring videos of the behavior chain they are willing to share. As the assessor, you may choose to extend the question probes asked (with the visual stimuli present). Given time constraints, if there are multiple OCBs, the therapist may pick and choose selective stimuli to use for further probing.
	Contriving situations to conduct brief exposures in the home and/or clinic. Prior to the assessment, you may ask a child and/or caregiver to contrive an exposure at home. For example, with ordering and arranging stimuli, you may ask a child to try moving a stimulus out of place and take note of whether they had to immediately move the stimulus back, exhibited distress, what they said, how they felt, etc. The brief exposure could also be done at the clinic if feasible and if the child is willing.

What Clinical Instruments Are Available and What Should You Choose?

Every clinician has their preferences when it comes to the use of standardized clinical assessments. If you are unfamiliar with OCB assessments, this list of suggestions and related links may be useful for you. Be mindful that this is not an exhaustive list and other options are available. Therapists can use these instruments to determine what categories of OCBs children and youth need assistance with.

- International OCD Foundation: Search this website for various assessment tools and resources, such as the Child OC Impact Scale–Revised (COIS-R; Piacentini et al., 2007).
- A recommended standardized instrument is the Children's Yale-Brown Obsessive Compulsive Scale (CY-BOCS; Goodman et al., 1986).
- *Here is a key reference for the CY-BOCS regarding its reliability and validity: Scahill, L., Riddle, M. A., McSwiggin-Hardin, M., Ort, S. I., King, R. A., Goodman, W. K., Cicchetti, D., & Leckman, J. F. (1997). Children's Yale-Brown Obsessive Compulsive Scale: reliability and validity. *Journal of the American Academy of Child and Adolescent Psychiatry*, 36(6), 844–852. https://doi.org/10.1097/00004583-199706000-00023

You may also want to ask questions like this one to gauge consumer satisfaction: "Overall, how satisfied were you with the effectiveness of therapy?" with 1 being not at all satisfied and 7 being very satisfied.

OCB Assessment in the RCT: Blended Clinical and Behavioral Assessment

Here, we present the step-by-step outline for conducting a blended clinical and behavioral assessment of OCBs that we used in the RCT. This is just one way to assess OCBs; you may use this as a guide or have your own assessment method. Below, we have outlined the steps followed in the RCT:

1. We had caregivers complete the Repetitive Behavior Scale – Revised (RBS-R; Bodfish et al., 1999; Appendix A). This is a 43-item caregiver rating measure. It is ideal to have caregivers complete all items, but if time constraints present themselves, ask them to complete the Sameness, Ritualistic, and Compulsive subscales (items 15 through 39).
2. When the RBS-R is completed, the clinician asked the responders about the endorsed items. For example, item 24 on the RBS-R states the following under the general title of Sleeping/Bedtime. The description is as follows:

Box 2.2   Item on RBS-R

SLEEPING / BEDTIME (Insists on certain pre-bedtime routines; Arranges items in the room "just so" prior to bedtime; Insists that certain items be present with him/her during sleep; Insists that another person be present prior to or during sleep).

The clinician may need to unpack the items further. *If there is a regimented routine, what does it consist of? What types of stimuli are involved? Who needs to be present while the child engages in the OCB and does this person need to engage in specific actions (e.g., give reassurance in a specific way)?*

At this point, you could inquire about related obsessions or wait until you shift over to your chosen standardized clinical assessment to gather information on obsessions and compulsions. You may also begin the process of ruling out behaviors that may have operant functions other than anxiety reduction. You also want to attend to developmental considerations (e.g., learning profile) and identify the level of the OCBs' interference. Take careful notes of all potential OCBs and descriptions of them (e.g., components involved, if a thought/obsession is present).

3. From the RBS-R, you have an idea of behaviors/general areas you would like to inquire about when moving to your standardized OCD assessment. In the RCT, after completing the RBS-R, we moved to the CY-BOCS. Given that the CY-BOCS has blank spaces in each section for miscellaneous items, any items that came up on the RBS-R were inserted into the appropriate section.

4. You may choose to use an **Obsessions and Compulsions Recording Template** (Appendix B), as we did in the RCT, at some point during the assessment. This may help obtain more information about obsessions and compulsions. As part of the template, there are suggested probes regarding obsessions and compulsions.

5. Many instruments like the CY-BOCS allow you to obtain information about variables such as duration, level of distress, resistance in performing the compulsion, and daily interference of OCBs in doing things at school and interacting with friends and family (Goodman et al., 1986). This is often rich information that helps a clinician form a clinical picture of each OCB and prioritize based on these variables. In the RCT, we used the CY-BOCS to gather this information.

6. After filling out the **Obsessions and Compulsions Recording Template** (Appendix B), we gathered more information about the topography of OCBs, their degree of interference, the desired post-treatment levels using the **Operational Definitions and Interference handout** (see Appendix C). In our experience, caregivers will use indicators like duration (or time it takes up each day) and interference in the child's and family members' lives. *How much does each OCB interfere with interacting with family and friends? Does it prevent the child from engaging in preferred/other activities? Are the OCBs getting in the way of flexibility in a family's daily routine?* These indicators are often part of a standardized assessment like the CY-BOCS (Goodman et al., 1986) but also should be considered as sessions progress when deciding (with the child and caregiver) which behaviors to focus on in treatment.

7. The **Operational Definitions and Interference** handout (Appendix C) allows you to list identified OCBs and the steps of each compulsion (e.g., steps of a routine) or what the compulsion consists of (e.g., a reassurance statement). You may want to group OCBs that occur in different settings but contain the same or a similar behavior into one OCB (e.g., sitting in the same seat in the car and at the dinner table) or list them as two separate OCBs.

As a clinician, you would involve the child and caregiver in discussing the compulsions and topographies of behavior. Stated differently, you attempt to capture all components or specific movements that make up the response and often comprise a behavioral chain (Martin & Pear, 2024). You may also want to note other behavioral characteristics such as duration, frequency, latency, or other behavioral dimensions. Last, you want to record the starting level (the baseline or pre-treatment level of the OCB) and the desired level (where you would like the OCB to be at post-treatment). This is needed for the **Caregiver Weekly Data Form** (Appendix D).

Suppose it is a regimented morning routine that an individual needs to follow. You would write down all the routine steps in the order that the child needs to perform them. Alternatively, think of repetitive reassurance seeking. It may be writing down the vocal reassurance requested by the child and, in some cases, the specific words that need to be strung together in a phrase (e.g., "Daddy is fine and will be home at 5 pm"). You may also want to record the duration of bouts of reassurance seeking or the approximate frequency (whichever makes sense for specific OCBs).

8. The last piece was putting together a caregiver data sheet to collect weekly data on OCBs. We completed this with information gathered from the child and caregiver. See Appendix D for a sample **Caregiver Weekly Data Form** with Likert scale questions, with 1 (representing desired post-treatment levels of OCBs) to 3 (partial improvement from pre-treatment levels) to 5 (pre-treatment levels of OCBs). A blank **Caregiver Weekly Data Form** has been provided in Appendix E. The **Operational Definitions and Interference** sheet may help formulate questions to guide data collection (Appendix C) and discuss the interference of OCBs. We collected caregiver weekly data in our RCT (Vause, Jaksic et al., 2020) to track the OCBs that we were targeting and those that remained in baseline. Using the caregiver data sheet and Stimulus Map (see activities in the Children's Workbook), you can assess the reduction in OCBs targeted in treatment.

General Acknowledgment of the Complexity of OCBs and Assessing Covert Behavior

A clinician may be unsure as to whether an OCB is maintained by anxiety reduction. However, if it is deemed interfering, Fb-CBT may be helpful. It allows for gradual response prevention of interfering compulsive behavior and teaching coping techniques. Specifically, children and youth who are not allowed to complete something or are not given access to a preferred person/stimulus may become upset, and coping strategies like counting, breathing, etc. may be helpful. It is important to note that it is also very difficult (or nearly impossible) to "prove" the anxiety component if the child is not able to verbalize it or does not show stable physiological sensations BUT has the need to order and arrange or handwash for long periods. Furthermore, it may be a "not just right" feeling or a fear of something bad happening that the child cannot verbalize. However, if the behavior is interfering, it is often worth putting the time and effort into Fb-CBT programming. In our experience, many children began to vocalize thoughts during treatment. We believe that it is to the client's benefit to treat a higher-order RRB in the OCD subset that is interfering and possibly anxiety-related than not to consider all treatment options in trying to reduce or alleviate an interfering compulsive behavior.

Satisfying Regulatory States

It is important to consider regulatory states and ensure you are attending to sensory/emotional regulation and what the child or youth needs.

For example, when a child presents with an OCB of sitting in the same seat, you may vary seats during treatment so the child can sit in their preferred seat a portion of the time. The goal is that they can be flexible with seating arrangements. As another example, allowing rearranging and ordering when it is not interfering and perhaps functional may help satisfy the need for internal sensory reinforcement. For example, the child may arrange a certain bin in their bedroom. Acknowledging what an individual needs from a function-based perspective and "choosing your battles" is necessary.

General Diagnostic Considerations for Professionals

In Chapter 1, we mentioned that challenges in self-awareness and introspection associated with autism may be barriers to children and youth vocalizing their thoughts. Further, a child's verbal ability, processing skills, cognitive processes, and executive functioning skills may contribute to a challenge in verbalizing obsessions. Also, if rapport building is not sufficient or a child feels uneasy or uncomfortable discussing thoughts, obsessions that are associated with compulsions may not emerge during assessment. Given these issues and others, both neurotypical and neurodiverse children often experience difficulties with obsession identification (APA, 2022). Suggestions are offered regarding using more concrete questions that may be helpful to the child or youth.

If diagnosis is in your scope of practice, here are some things you may want to consider when conducting your diagnostic workup of OCD:

1. Children may struggle with describing obsessions and may vocalize thoughts related to some compulsions and not others. You may attempt a more concrete line of questioning (e.g., Franklin et al., 2019) or revisit specific compulsions later to inquire about thoughts.
2. You may want to consider the consistency of physiological sensations (e.g., increased redness of the face, sweatiness) if the compulsion is prevented. This may be accomplished through a conversation and/or behavioral observation. Are these observed signs of anxiety or agitation consistent before the compulsion or when prevented from engaging in it? If a child or youth is unable to verbalize the obsession, physiological sensations may give you some information regarding tension and anxiety symptoms present prior to the compulsion.

3. In addition to gathering information on compulsions, check avoidance behaviors (e.g., avoiding restrooms to prevent becoming contaminated; March & Mulle, 1998).
4. A medical history should be conducted to determine if other complexities or conditions need to be considered, such as Pediatric Acute-onset Neuropathic Disorders Associated with Streptococcus (PANS; Franklin et al., 2019).
5. Check if there is a familial history of OCD and related disorders in the immediate and extended family.
6. In addition to conducting a standardized assessment and observational measures, refer to diagnostic criteria of OCD including duration (more than one hour per day of engaging in OCBs) and clinically significant distress in various areas of everyday functioning (APA, 2022).
7. Consider psychiatric, neurodevelopmental, and other conditions that may better represent symptom presentation. For example, regimented ways of eating or dressing may be associated with social anxiety disorder and certain behaviors associated with exaggerated fears may represent a specific phobia. Other disorders mentioned earlier include skin picking and tic disorders. Intense preoccupations about certain topics (e.g., space) and lower-level RRBs may be subsumed under autism.

We understand that many professionals (e.g., general practitioners, pediatricians, psychiatrists, and psychologists) have extensive training in this decision-making process. We offer these points as considerations that may be helpful when examining whether an OCD diagnosis should be given. These are just a few considerations in unpacking symptoms and reflecting on whether compulsive behaviors are subsumed under OCD or may be assigned a separate diagnosis. A separate diagnosis may be helpful when considering medication or accessing services or funding.

References

American Psychiatric Association. (2022). *Diagnostic and statistical manual of mental disorders* (5th ed., text rev.). https://doi.org/10.1176/appi.books.9780890425787

Bodfish, J. W., Symons, F. J., & Lewis, M. H. (1999). *The Repetitive Behavior Scale: Test manual*. Western Carolina Center Research Reports.

Bodfish, J. W., Symons, F. J., Parker, D. E., & Lewis, M. H. (2000). Varieties of repetitive behavior in autism: Comparisons to mental retardation. *Journal of Autism and Developmental Disorders, 30*, 237–243. https://doi.org/10.1177/1362361311414066

Boyd, B. A., McDonough, S. G., & Bodfish, J. W. (2012). Evidence-based behavioral interventions for repetitive behaviors in autism. *Journal of Autism and Developmental Disorders, 42*(6), 1236–1248. https://doi.org/10.1007/s10803-011-1284-z

Fisher, W. W., Piazza, C. C., Bowman, L. G., & Amari, A. (1996). Integrating caregiver report with systematic choice assessment to enhance reinforcer identification. *American Journal of Mental Retardation, 101*(1), 15–25.

Franklin, M. E., Freeman, J. B., & March, J. S. (2019). *Treating OCD in children and adolescents: A cognitive-behavioral approach.* Guilford Press.

Goodman, W. K., Price, L. H., Rasmussen, S. A., Riddle, M. A., & Rapoport, J. L. (1986). *Children's yale-brown obsessive compulsive scale (CY-BOCS).* National Institutes of Mental Health (public domain).

March, J. S., & Mulle, K. (1998). *OCD in children and adolescents: A cognitive-behavioral treatment manual.* Guilford Press.

Martin, G., & Pear, J. J. (2024). *Behavior modification: What is it and how to do it* (12th ed.). Routledge.

Mirenda, P., Smith, I. M., Vaillancourt, T., Georgiades, S., Duku, E., Szatmari, P., Bryson, S., Fombonne, E., Roberts, W., Volden, J., Waddell, C., Zwaigenbaum, L., & Pathways in ASD Study Team. (2010). Validating the Repetitive Behavior Scale-Revised in young children with autism spectrum disorder. *Journal of Autism and Developmental Disorders, 40*(12), 1521–1530. https://doi.org/10.1007/s10803-010-1012-0

Oar, E. L., Johnco, C., & Ollendick, T. H. (2017). Cognitive behavioral therapy for anxiety and depression in children and adolescents. *The Psychiatric Clinics of North America, 40*(4), 661–674. https://doi.org/10.1016/j.psc.2017.08.002

Piacentini, J., Langley, A., & Roblek, T. (2007). *Overcoming childhood OCD: A cognitive behavioral treatment program.* Oxford University Press.

Scahill, L., Riddle, M. A., McSwiggin-Hardin, M., Ort, S. I., King, R. A., Goodman, W. K., Cicchetti, D., & Leckman, J. F. (1997). Children's Yale-Brown Obsessive Compulsive Scale: Reliability and validity. *Journal of the American Academy of Child and Adolescent Psychiatry, 36*(6), 844–852. https://doi.org/10.1097/00004583-199706000-00023

Vause, T., Jaksic, H., Neil, N., Frijters, J. C., Jackiewicz, G., & Feldman, M. (2020). Functional behavior-based cognitive-behavioral therapy for obsessive compulsive behavior in children with autism spectrum disorder: A randomized controlled trial. *Journal of Autism and Developmental Disorders, 50*(7), 2375–2388. https://doi.org/10.1007/s10803-018-3772-x

Appendix A

Repetitive Behavior Scale – Revised

Reprinted with permission from authors Bodfish, Symons, and Lewis.

INSTRUCTIONS: Please rate this person's behavior by reading each of the items listed and then choosing the score that best describes how much of a problem the item is for the person. Be sure to read and score all items listed. Make your ratings based on your observations and interactions with the person over the last month. Use the definitions in the box given to score each item.

> 0 = behavior *does not occur*
> 1 = behavior occurs and is a *mild* problem
> 2 = behavior occurs and is a *moderate* problem
> 3 = behavior occurs and is a *severe* problem

When deciding on a score for each item, consider: (a) *how frequently the behavior occurs* (e.g., weekly versus hourly), (b) *how difficult it is to interrupt the behavior* (e.g., can be easily redirected versus becomes distressed if interrupted) and (c) *how much the behavior interferes* with ongoing events (e.g., easy to ignore or overlook versus very disruptive).

Name:_____ ID#: _____

Gender: ☐ Female ☐ Male   **Date of Birth**: ___ / ___ / _____

Today's Date:___/___/_____Informant's Name:_____

I. Stereotyped Behavior Subscale

DEFINITION: apparently purposeless movements or actions that are repeated in a similar manner

1	WHOLE BODY (Body rocking, Body swaying)	0	1	2	3
2	HEAD (Rolls Head, Nods Head, Turns Head)	0	1	2	3
3	HAND/FINGER (Flaps hands, Wiggles or flicks fingers, Claps hands, Waves or shakes hand or arm)	0	1	2	3
4	LOCOMOTION (Turns in circle(s), Whirls, Jumps, Bounces)	0	1	2	3
5	OBJECT USAGE (Spins or twirls objects, Twiddles or slaps or throws objects, Lets objects fall out of hands)	0	1	2	3
6	SENSORY (Covers eyes, Looks closely or gazes at hands or objects, Covers ears, Smells or sniffs items, Rubs surfaces)	0	1	2	3

> 0 = behavior *does not occur*
> 1 = behavior occurs and is a *mild* problem
> 2 = behavior occurs and is a *moderate* problem
> 3 = behavior occurs and is a *severe* problem

II. Self-Injurious Behavior Subscale

DEFINITION: movement or actions that have the potential to cause redness, bruising, or other injury to the body, and that are repeated in a similar manner

7	HITS SELF WITH BODY PART (Hits or slaps head, face, or other body area)	0	1	2	3
8	HITS SELF AGAINST SURFACE OR OBJECT (Hits or bangs head or other body part on table, floor, or other surface)	0	1	2	3
9	HITS SELF WITH OBJECT (Hits or bangs head or other body area with objects)	0	1	2	3
10	BITES SELF (Bites hand, wrist, arm, lips, or tongue)	0	1	2	3
11	PULLS (Pulls hair or skin)	0	1	2	3
12	RUBS OR SCRATCHES SELF (Rubs or scratches marks on arms, leg, face, or torso)	0	1	2	3
13	INSERTS FINGER OR OBJECT (Eye-poking, Ear-poking)	0	1	2	3
14	SKIN PICKING (Picks at skin on face, hands, arms, legs, or torso)	0	1	2	3

III.   Compulsive Behavior Subscale

DEFINITION: behavior that is repeated and is performed according to a rule, or involves things being done "just so"

15	ARRANGING / ORDERING (Arranges certain objects in a particular pattern or place; Need for things to be even or symmetrical)	0	1	2	3
16	COMPLETENESS (Must have doors opened or closed; Takes all items out of a container or area)	0	1	2	3
17	WASHING / CLEANING (Excessively cleans certain body parts; Picks at lint or loose threads)	0	1	2	3
18	CHECKING (Repeatedly checks doors, windows, drawers, appliances, clocks, locks, etc.)	0	1	2	3
19	COUNTING (Counts items or objects; Counts to a certain number or in a certain way)	0	1	2	3
20	HOARDING/SAVING (Collects, hoards, or hides specific items)	0	1	2	3
21	REPEATING (Need to repeat routine events; In / out door, up / down from chair, clothing on/off)	0	1	2	3
22	TOUCH / TAP (Need to touch, tap, or rub items, surfaces, or people)	0	1	2	3

```
0 = behavior does not occur
1 = behavior occurs and is a mild problem
2 = behavior occurs and is a moderate problem
3 = behavior occurs and is a severe problem
```

IV.   Ritualistic Behavior Subscale

DEFINITION: performing activities of daily living in a similar manner

23	EATING / MEALTIME (Strongly prefers/insists on eating/ drinking only certain things; Eats or drinks items in a set order; Insists that meal related items are arranged in a certain way)	0	1	2	3
24	SLEEPING / BEDTIME (Insists on certain pre-bedtime routines; Arranges items in room "just so" prior to bedtime; Insists that certain items be present with him/her during sleep; Insists that another person be present prior to or during sleep)	0	1	2	3
25	SELF-CARE – BATHROOM AND DRESSING (Insists on specific order of activities or tasks related to using the bathroom, to washing, showering, bathing or dressing; Arranges items in a certain way in the bathroom or insists that bathroom items not be moved; Insists on wearing certain clothing items)	0	1	2	3
26	TRAVEL / TRANSPORTATION (Insists on taking certain routes/paths; Must sit in specific location in vehicles; Insists that certain items be present during travel, e.g., toy or material; Insists on seeing or touching certain things or places during travel such as a sign or store)	0	1	2	3
27	PLAY / LEISURE (Insists on certain play activities; Follows a rigid routine during play / leisure; Insists that certain items be present/available during play/leisure; Insists that other persons do certain things during play)	0	1	2	3
28	COMMUNICATION / SOCIAL INTERACTIONS (Repeats same topic(s) during social interactions; Repetitive questioning; Insists on certain topics of conversation; Insists that others say certain things or respond in certain ways during interactions)	0	1	2	3

V.   Sameness Behavior Subscale

DEFINITION: resistance to change, insisting that things stay the same

29	Insists that things remain in the same place(s) (e.g., toys, supplies, furniture, pictures, etc.)	0	1	2	3
30	Objects to visiting new places	0	1	2	3
31	Becomes upset if interrupted in what he/she is doing	0	1	2	3
32	Insists on walking in a particular pattern (e.g., straight line)	0	1	2	3
33	Insists on sitting at the same place	0	1	2	3
34	Dislikes changes in appearance or behavior of the people around him/her	0	1	2	3
35	Insists on using a particular door	0	1	2	3
36	Likes the same CD, tape, record or piece of music played continually; Likes same movie / video or part of movie / video	0	1	2	3
37	Resists changing activities; Difficulty with transitions	0	1	2	3
38	Insists on same routine, household, school, or work schedule every day	0	1	2	3
39	Insists that specific things take place at specific times	0	1	2	3

> 0 = behavior *does not occur*
> 1 = behavior occurs and is a *mild* problem
> 2 = behavior occurs and is a *moderate* problem
> 3 = behavior occurs and is a *severe* problem

VI.   Restricted Behavior Subscale

DEFINITION: Limited range of focus, interest, or activity

40	Fascination, preoccupation with one subject or activity (e.g., trains, computers, weather, dinosaurs)	0	1	2	3
41	Strongly attached to one specific object	0	1	2	3
42	Preoccupation with part(s) of object rather than the whole object (e.g., buttons on clothes, wheels on toy cars)	0	1	2	3
43	Fascination, preoccupation with movement / things that move (e.g., fans, clocks)	0	1	2	3

Scoring Summary

1. **Number of subscale items endorsed**: number of items in a sub-scale rated 1, 2, or 3
2. **Total subscale score**: sum of the ratings for all of the items in a subscale
3. **Overall number of items endorsed**: sum of the "Number of sub-scale items endorsed"
4. **Overall score**: sum of the "Total subscale scores"

Subscale	Number of subscale items endorsed	Total subscale score
I. Stereotyped Behavior		
II. Self-injurious Behavior		
III. Compulsive Behavior		
IV. Ritualistic Behavior		
V. Sameness Behavior		
VI. Restricted Behavior		

Overall number of items endorsed	Overall Score

References for RBS-R

Bodfish, J.W., Symons, F.J., Parker, D.E., & Lewis, M.H. (2000). Varieties of repetitive behavior in autism. *Journal of Autism and Developmental Disabilities*, 30, 237–243.
Bodfish, J.W., Symons, F.J., Lewis, M.H. (1999). *The Repetitive Behavior Scale*. Western Carolina Center Research Reports.

Appendix B

Obsession and Compulsion Recording Template

Name: _____   Date: _____

OBSESSIONS	COMPULSIONS
Sample Probes: • Why do you have to [compulsion]? • What do you think about right before [compulsion]?"	**Sample Probes:** • How would you feel if you were prevented from doing [compulsion]? With this question, you may be able to draw out the obsession and/or distress associated with not doing the compulsion.
1.	1.
2.	2.
3.	3.
4.	4.
5.	5.
6.	6.
7.	7.
8.	8.
9.	9.
10.	10.

Appendix C

Operational Definitions and Interference Form

Child/Caregiver: _____   Date: _____

Gathering Information and Assessing Interference of OCBs *How much does each OCB interfere with interacting with family and friends? Does it prevent the child or youth from engaging in preferred/other activities? Are the OCBs creating inflexibility in the daily routine and impacting the child and family's lives? (Goodman et al., 1986)*	Is it deemed interfering?	Would the child be distressed if they could not perform the compulsion?
Obsession #1: Compulsion #1 (List all steps, if applicable): Starting Level: Desired Level:	Yes No	Yes No
Obsession #2: Compulsion #2 (List all steps, if applicable): Starting Level: Desired Level:	Yes No	Yes No
Obsession #3: Compulsion #3 (List all steps, if applicable): Starting Level: Desired Level:	Yes No	Yes No
Obsession #4: Compulsion #4 (List all steps, if applicable): Starting Level: Desired Level: Obsession #5: Compulsion #5 (List all steps, if applicable): Starting Level: Desired Level:	Yes No Yes No	Yes No Yes No

Note: Starting Level is where the OCB is at pre-treatment. Desired Level is where the child/caregiver would like the OCB post-treatment.

Appendix D

Sample Caregiver Weekly Data Form

Caregiver Check-in Form					
Informant (first and last name):					
Date (mm/dd/yy):					
1. Throughout the day, how many times did J need to touch one side of his body after touching the other?					
N/A☐	1☐	2☐	3☐	4☐	5☐
	0 times		10 times		20 times
2. This morning, how many times did J ask for reassurance about Dad?					
N/A☐	1☐	2☐	3☐	4☐	5☐
Dad didn't leave house	0 times		5 times		10+ times
3. Throughout the day, how long could J wait before moving Lego items back?					
N/A☐	1☐	2☐	3☐	4☐	5☐
No access to Lego	0 minutes		2 minutes		30 seconds
4. Throughout the day, how many times did J tell on his brother or dad?					
N/A☐	1☐	2☐	3☐	4☐	5☐
	0 times	1 time	2–3 times	4 times	5+ times
5. Throughout the day, how long did J handwash?					
N/A☐	1☐	2☐	3☐	4☐	5☐
	1 minute		5 minutes		10 minutes

6. Throughout the day, how many times did J use preventative measures to avoid germs (e.g., shirt over face, foot for garbage, avoid touching door knobs)?

N/A☐	1☐	2☐	3☐	4☐	5☐
	0 times	1–5 times	6–10 times	11–15 times	16+ times

7. Did J have to complete his entire bedtime routine tonight (i.e., pajamas, snack, sister to bed, read story, say prayers, hold his teddy and dolphin, and have blanket cover ears?)

N/A☐	1☐	2☐	3☐	4☐	5☐
	Flexible in changing 3+ items		Flexible in changing 1 item		Yes, he did

8. During meals, Did J have to sit in the same seat today?

N/A☐	1☐	2☐	3☐	4☐	5☐
	No, he didn't		Sat in new seat for 1 meal		Yes, he did

Comments:

Note: These are simply examples based on OCB caregiver data from the RCT. For any given item, feel free to offer all five anchors or fewer, depending on variables such as the behavior dimension, caregiver feasibility, etc. Caregivers are then encouraged to use their best judgment when scoring OCBs on the scales provided.

Appendix E

Blank Caregiver Weekly Data Form

Caregiver Data Sheet					
Name of Data Collector:					
Date:					
1.					
N/A	1	2	3	4	5
2.					
N/A	1	2	3	4	5
3.					
N/A	1	2	3	4	5
4.					
N/A	1	2	3	4	5
5.					
N/A	1	2	3	4	5

Chapter 3

Functional Assessment and Function-Based Intervention

Functional Approach

One of the unique aspects of functional behavior-based cognitive behavioral therapy (Fb-CBT) is that it combines principles and strategies of both cognitive behavior therapy (CBT) and applied behavior analysis (ABA). This chapter will focus on the ABA components. In a functional behavior-analytic approach to obsessive-compulsive behavior (OCB), behavior is viewed as functional for certain contexts because of the contingencies involved. A contingency is the temporal relationship between a behavior and a consequence and is often stated as an "if-then" rule. *If* you brush your teeth, *then* we will read a bedtime story. *If* you touch the hot burner, *then* you will feel pain. These consequences influence behavior, making it more or less likely to occur in the same or similar contexts.

Both respondent and operant contingencies are important in the formation and maintenance of OCBs (Guertin et al., 2022; Mowrer, 1951). Neutral stimuli begin to elicit fear responses through classical conditioning, where a neutral stimulus (such as a specific situation or object) and an aversive or fear-inducing stimulus (like a loud noise) become associated through repeated pairings. For example, if a person has a fear-inducing experience, such as choking on a carrot, they can become fearful of eating carrots. Carrots, which were initially neutral stimuli, now being paired with fear become conditioned stimuli for fear and anxiety. Through the higher-order conditioning and relational learning processes, other things can also become conditioned stimuli for fear, such as other vegetables or all hard foods. This process can aid our understanding of how anxiety-based obsessions and compulsions initially develop.

In Chapter 1, we discuss how obsessions and environmental events can act as an **establishing operation** (EO; Martin & Pear, 2024) by

DOI: 10.4324/9781003410126-3

eliciting distress. This then increases the value of anxiety relief as a reinforcer and increases the likelihood of behavior that reduces distress (compulsions). Compulsions are maintained by negative reinforcement; when a child performs a compulsion, the distress is reduced. This increases the likelihood that the child will engage in the compulsion again in similar contexts. They also might engage in avoidance behavior (like avoiding the situation or object) to prevent or reduce internal states of distress. For the child who has developed a fear of eating carrots, vegetables, and other hard foods might engage in ritualized eating which involves avoiding those foods as well as present with compulsions that reduce distress when presented with those foods such as cutting them in a certain way, requesting that parents boil them, or repeatedly asking for reassurance (Guertin et al., 2022). When avoidance behavior and compulsions successfully prevent or remove the aversive stimulus, it negatively reinforces the avoidance response. This strengthens the tendency to avoid the feared stimulus in the future and perform the compulsions.

Functions of OCBs

There are two functions of operant behavior: positive reinforcement and negative reinforcement. **Positive reinforcement** (also known as access functions; left side of Figure 3.1) involves behavior that produces an environmental event that subsequently increases the likelihood of that behavior under the same or similar conditions. When a child gets or accesses something as a result of their behavior and there is an increase of that behavior in the future, that is a positive reinforcement function. For example, if a child asks for a snack using "please" and the parent gives them the snack only when the child says "please," then the child is more likely to use "please" in the future. In a positive reinforcement contingency, consequences can be various things, such as interactions with preferred people, access to preferred activities, or sensory stimulation (i.e., a pleasant sensation). For something to act as a reinforcer, it simply must be something that when delivered as a consequence for a particular behavior, there is an increased likelihood that the behavior will be repeated.

When the behavior serves to escape or avoid something, that is a **negative reinforcement** function (right side of Figure 3.1). In a negative reinforcement function, the behavior terminates or postpones an environmental event resulting in an increased likelihood of that behavior under the same

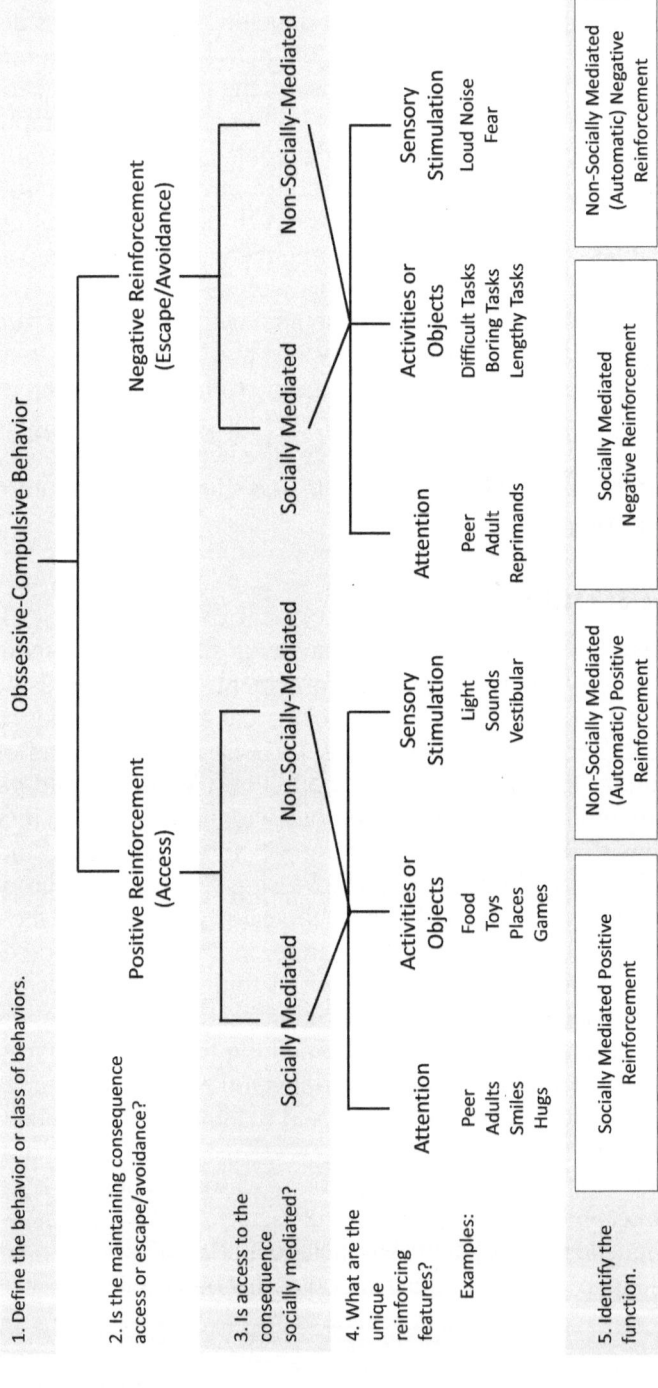

Figure 3.1 The functions of behavior.

or similar conditions. For example, a child puts on their seatbelt when they enter the car, and the seatbelt chime stops dinging. The child is more likely to buckle their seatbelt immediately to avoid the sound in the future. Like positive reinforcers, negative reinforcers can take different forms such as the removal of difficult or boring activities, avoiding non-preferred people, or removing uncomfortable sensory stimulation or distressing thoughts like in the case of OCBs. For example, a child may engage in a compulsion (e.g., handwashing) to alleviate a distressing obsession (e.g., fear of getting germs on themselves that leads to getting sick).

Positive reinforcement and negative reinforcement can be **non-socially mediated** or **socially mediated** (row 3 in Figure 3.1). Non-socially mediated can also be referred to as direct access or automatic reinforcement. Here, the consequence is directly produced by the behavior. For example, washing hands eliminates the thought of contamination, or opening the blinds provides access to sunlight. Other times, consequences are produced through the behavior being mediated by another individual. They produced desired outcomes through the actions of another. For example, expressing fears about speaking in class results in an alternative assignment from the teacher or asking for reassurance about marks on your body to a caregiver results in them giving a Band-Aid.

Non-Socially Mediated Functions of OCB

Negative Reinforcement (to Escape)

Non-socially mediated negative reinforcement (also known as escape from sensory stimulation) is the most commonly thought of function when addressing OCBs. Typically, compulsive behavior serves the function of reducing anxiety and removing anxiety-inducing stimuli (e.g., dirty hands; items not lined up). Conditioned internal (thoughts and obsessions) or external (items, settings, events) stimuli elicit anxiety and distress, and by performing the compulsive behavior, there is a reduction in the individual's internal distress, and this reduction in distress and removal of anxiety stimuli increases the likelihood that the individual will perform the behavior in the same or similar conditions. An example from one of our Fb-CBT groups occurred in an 8-year-old who needed to sit in the same seat during car rides (Guertin et al., 2022). When asked to sit in other seats, she would cry and yell, stating, "No, I cannot do that." This was reportedly interfering with daily family outings. During initial assessments, she did not express obsessions or thoughts surrounding the behavior and the behavior appeared to serve an automatic function (i.e., liking the feeling of a particular seat). Later in treatment, she began to express harm to self-related obsessions because she voiced that the shoes she wore to a funeral touched the other seats. In addition to preferring a particular seat, sitting in the same seat resulted in relief from anxiety as she avoided the "poisonous" seats.

Non-socially mediated escape may also occur to avoid or terminate other events, such as social interactions, activities, and external sensory stimulation. An example of a non-socially meditated escape occurred with a child who displayed repeated checking behavior reporting that he needed to ensure things were "where they were supposed to be" and that they were safe. He was particularly concerned about the safety of structures he had made from LEGO® building blocks. This behavior regularly occurred in multiple contexts including less preferred social ones. Checking on the safety of items likely served a negative reinforcement function by reducing distress associated with fears around the safety of his items. Additionally, the checking involved him physically removing himself from the social context and producing direct escape from the social context.

Positive Reinforcement (to Access)

OCB may serve a positive reinforcement function that is non-socially mediated, this is also called automatic positive reinforcement or access to sensory stimulation. These behaviors are assumed to produce their own reinforcement through an unspecified process, such as through altering or maintaining states of sensory arousal. One participant in our groups (Adam) displayed ordering and straightening of objects (Vause et al., 2017) in his bed, including slippers, items on his headboard, and stuffed animals. He expressed no thoughts or obsessions related to the ordering but would repeatedly display overt signs of distress (e.g., excessive crying) if ordering and arranging were interrupted. It was hypothesized that the behavior was access to sensory reinforcement. Other studies which conducted experimental functional analysis on topographically similar behavior also arrived at similar functions, finding arranging and ordering in youth with autism was non-socially mediated reinforcement (Rodriguez et al., 2012). Chapter 1 highlights how children with autism and neurotypical school-age children often have difficulty communicating the thoughts and sensations that pair with their compulsions, making it difficult for clinicians to determine whether OCBs serve anxiety relief functions, such as a "not just right feeling," in addition to positive reinforcement or sensory functions (DSM-5-TR; American Psychiatric Association [APA], 2022). Reducing or eliminating behavior that serves this function may not always be a socially valid treatment goal. Autistic self-advocates note concerns caused by reducing these stereotypic or "stimming" behaviors as they may serve a comfort or self-regulatory function (Lynch, 2019). Clinicians should ensure that sensory needs are fulfilled with replacement behavior. In the case of Adam, he could have a bin to rearrange similar stuffed animals throughout the day as a replacement behavior. Alternatives could also be arranging other items that are preferred and discussed with the child.

Socially Mediated Functions of OCB

Repetitive behavior in autism and related disorders can also serve socially mediated functions. Socially mediated positive reinforcement refers to reinforcement that occurs via another person. In a positive reinforcement contingency, behavior is strengthened through the addition of a stimulus facilitated by another person. Examples of this might include access to praise, adult or peer attention, preferred activities, objects, or privileges. In a negative reinforcement context behavior is strengthened through the removal or avoidance of an aversive stimulus via another individual. Examples might include avoiding or escaping difficult tasks, boring tasks, easy tasks, physical demands, or non-preferred activities or people.

Negative Reinforcement (to Escape)

Socially mediated escape or socially mediated negative reinforcement is a commonly identified function among the children who participated in our treatment program. One example occurred with an 8-year-old boy (Maxim) who repeatedly erased and rewrote words during writing tasks throughout homework. Typically, homework was completed with the supervision of a parent. The child had some difficulty describing thoughts surrounding the behavior but did describe needing to print letters so that they were "just right." There were reported support needs with pre-academic tasks, and when observing we noted that when he repeatedly erased and rewrote words, the parent sometimes reduced the expectations (expecting fewer words or sheets to be completed), terminated the homework task, or assisted by acting as a scribe for the child. In this way, the child escaped the difficult or lengthy task through the parents' actions.

Positive Reinforcement (to Access)

OCBs which result in socially mediated access often occur through the form of reassurance seeking. The child asks repeated questions about their safety, contamination, rituals and routines, or things being "just right," and their parent replies. An example of socially mediated access occurred with an 11-year-old boy who participated in our Fb-CBT group who displayed repeated rubbing of his mother's arm and head. Initially, this behavior was captured in the touching, tapping, and rubbing portion of the OCB assessment, but our observations indicated that this behavior resulted in access to conversation and attention from his mother. Later in treatment, he verbalized that this behavior primarily served to gain his mother's attention.

Another participant, Michael, repeatedly sought reassurance from his mother about germs and getting sick and would ask his mother if he would catch germs. We found that Michael was likely to seek reassurance when he was around others who were sick, as well as at mealtimes, leading us to hypothesize a socially mediated access to attention function. It was also clear that this behavior was associated with thoughts around becoming sick, and reassurance-seeking increased when others in the household were sick, suggesting it also served an automatic negative reinforcement function to escape from anxiety. The treatment for this case is detailed later.

Multiple Functions

Numerous studies have shown that behavior can and often does serve multiple functions (Love et al., 2009; Reese et al., 2003). Behavior may be maintained by multiple reinforcers separately or by the interaction between reinforcers (Hanley et al., 2014; Slaton et al., 2017). For example, a tantrum may result in escape from a social context and access to parental attention. Behavior maintained by a single function may often be addressed with one intervention, whereas multiply controlled behavior usually requires a variety of elements and potentially differing interventions for each specific EO and functional reinforcer. For example, parents will often describe multiple EOs working at the same time; the parent turned off a movie and asked the child to go do their homework. The behavior that occurs, such as whining, refusal, and throwing items, results in multiple reinforcers including access to the movie and terminating the demand. Recent work has demonstrated the utility of assessing and treating behavior using synthesized contingencies, such as this (that is multiple EOs, multiple reinforcers, and multiple topographies of behavior; Slaton & Hanley, 2018). Further synthesized contingencies might be more reflective of typical home, school, and community environments. Children often escape difficult tasks to some activity, such as toys, tablets, or other tangible activities but rarely escape to "nothing."

In our experience with OCBs, they can and often serve multiple functions. For example, these behaviors might serve both an anxiety reduction function (e.g., negative reinforcement from sensory stimulation) and a socially mediated function (e.g., access to attention), such as in the case of Michael, whose reassurance seeking was related to fears around germs and illness as well as gaining attention from his mother. If the goal is a meaningful behavior change, it may not always be necessary to identify if a response has a single operant function or if it is maintained by more than one reinforcer, or the interaction between them. Because our treatment package involves a multicomponent approach addressing both the non-social and socially mediated functions of OCB, we would expect treatment effects whether or not the behavior is maintained by automatic negative reinforcement and/or by socially mediated functions as both are being addressed.

Another of our participants, Abigail, a 7-year-old, had several OCBs related to sitting in the same seat, including at the dinner table, and while watching TV in her living room. During initial assessments, she did not articulate thoughts surrounding why she sat in her preferred seats. Our functional assessments suggested that sitting in one spot in the living room had a tangible function; that is, non-socially mediated access to the best view of the television. As the group progressed, Abigail revealed that she sat in a particular seat while watching TV to avoid the recliner. Sitting in the recliner was associated with general fears of bad things happening to her, suggesting it was also maintained by non-socially mediated escape from anxiety.

The Functional Assessment Process

Functional behavioral assessment (FBA) is the generic term describing the process of identifying environmental variables that predict and

Table 3.1 Functional Behavior Assessment Steps

Description	Assessing Function	Summary of Findings
A detailed, precise description of the behavior, or classes and sequences of behavior that occur together	Identification of environmental variables that influence behavior including the setting events and antecedents that predict behavior and the consequences that maintain the behavior.	Development of a hypothesis statement that describes the function of the behavior.

maintain behavior before intervention. The purpose is to gather information that can be used to develop a function-based intervention to replace challenging behavior with adaptive skills that obtain the same or similar reinforcement.

Table 3.1 shows the steps of a functional behavior assessment. The process is supported by data-based decision-making, information is gathered through indirect observations, direct observations, and functional analysis.

Although there is no set description of the particular skills needed to conduct a functional behavior assessment and create behavior intervention plans, we assume that users will have some basic training and experience in the practice and theory of applied behavior analysis and behavior interventions to support individuals with interfering behavior.

Description

The first step of the process is identifying behavior that will serve as the target of the functional assessment and intervention strategies. In your clinical assessment, you will have identified an initial list of interfering OCBs you will be targeting during treatment, and we have provided resources to develop operational definitions (see Chapter 2). Defining OCBs in an observable measurable way is an important component of a functional behavior assessment. These definitions promote communication between therapists, caregivers, and children and reliable measurement of the OCBs. These definitions also support functional behavior intervention planning, and exposure and response prevention.

Although we discuss developing operational definitions during initial assessments in Chapter 2, you might encounter information during sessions that result in the need to refine definitions.

In addition to defining the behavior in observable terms, clinicians should also seek to identify precursors to OCBs. Precursors are responses that tend to occur immediately before OCBs, for example, an individual may say, "I need to fix this," before engaging in arranging or ordering. To identify precursors, consider questions such as, "Are there behaviors that seem to indicate the [OCB] is about to occur?" and "Does [OCB] appear in clusters or bursts with other behavior?"

Once an OCB has been identified and defined, traditionally the next step is to quantify the level of responding. Ways to measure and quantify the level of behavior are detailed elsewhere (Cooper et al., 2019), and these can include frequency, duration, or percentage of occurrence measures. These data serve as a baseline assessment. (See Chapter 2 for more information gathered during initial assessments.) During our research studies, we gathered information on the frequency or duration of OCBs via caregiver rating scales, ranging from 1 (desired posttreatment levels of OCBs) to 3 (partial improvement from pretreatment levels) to 5 (pretreatment levels of OCBs). Chapter 2 provides sample caregiver tracking sheets which can be modified for use.

Assessing Function

With a clear understanding of what the OCB looks like, you now need to collect information that identifies the environmental events maintaining the OCB including the immediate antecedents that predict when behavior will and will not occur, setting events that influence the probability of the OCB occurring, and the consequences that maintain the OCB. This allows you to generate a hypothesis about the function of the behavior. Based on your hypothesis, you can then select treatment strategies for the behavior that addresses the function.

Antecedents

Antecedents refer to environmental events that occur immediately before the OCB. They are immediate predictors of the OCB and can include when and where the OCB occurs, along with who and what activities it occurs in the presence of. Antecedents signal the availability of consequences, letting them know that their behavior will result in reinforcing consequences. For example, when a caregiver is present, repetitive question asking will be reinforced with answers to those questions, but not when the caregiver is absent. As with identifying precursors, the OCB News activity (in the Children's Workbook) can be a valuable source of information on antecedents. This activity asks participants about the who, what, where, and when of their OCBs. In some instances, the OCB may occur whenever an activity is presented. For example, the participant may wash their hands when any dirt or mark is present on themselves. In other cases, the combination of these aspects may be important, that is, OCB may occur when certain people are present and when engaging in a particular activity. For example, one of our group participants had to sit in a particular seat only at home during dinnertime. Some antecedents may be private events, such as intraverbal rules or obsessions, that make them more difficult to identify. As mentioned, it may take time for the child to be able to externally verbalize these covert behaviors.

Box 3.1   Questions to Consider When Identifying Antecedents

1. What happens immediately before the OCB? Can you describe the situation in detail?
2. Where does the behavior typically occur? Is there a specific location where the behavior is more likely to happen?
3. How do others interact with the child before the OCB occurs?
4. What activities or tasks are taking place before the OCB?
5. What kinds of demands or requests are made before the OCB?
6. Are there any changes in the environment (noise, lighting, or other sensory conditions) before the OCB occurs?
7. Are there specific objects or items present that might trigger the OCB?

Setting Events

Setting events are aspects of a person's environment that do not always occur immediately before or after the OCB but affect the probability of an OCB being performed. They may be internal or external to the individual. For example, if a setting is loud, if there are large crowds, if there are novel or unpredictable schedule changes, these events may increase the value of escape from a setting as a reinforcer. Setting events can also be physiological, such as pain, lack of sleep, or menstruation. Physical discomfort may increase the value of escape from difficult tasks as a reinforcer. Lack of contact with peers or adults may increase the value of attention as a reinforcer. In more precise terms, the events may act as EOs and are environmental events that affect the reinforcing effectiveness of a consequence and alter the frequency of behavior that has previously resulted in that consequence (Michael, 1993).

Box 3.2   Questions to Consider When Identifying Setting Events

8. Does the OCB consistently occur (or not occur) during certain periods of the day?
9. Is the person on any prescription medications, what are the effects and side effects?
10. Are there sleep-related issues that might affect behavior?
11. Are there eating or food-related issues that might affect behavior?
12. Are there periods or activities when the OCB is very likely to occur?
13. Are there patterns related to people or staff associated with the OCB?

Consequences

Consequences are events that follow the OCB, or what the person experiences as a result of their behavior. Like antecedents, consequences alter the likelihood of behavior occurring through their reinforcement and punishing functions. Antecedents, however, alter the current likelihood of behavior, while consequences influence the future likelihood. By analyzing the consequences that follow an OCB, you can hypothesize the function that the behavior serves for the individual.

Assessments

There are three main approaches to assessing function: indirect (interviews, rating scales, checklists), descriptive (direct observation in natural conditions), and functional analysis (systematic manipulation of environmental events). Often, a combination of one or more is used during the assessment process.

Indirect Assessments

Indirect approaches are those in which there is no direct observation of behavior and can include rating scales, questionnaires, and interviews (Paclawskyj et al., 2000). In our published work, we used the Questions About Behavior Function (QABF; Matson & Vollmer, 1995), an indirect assessment of behavioral function that consists of 25 items. Caregivers familiar with the individual rate each item, and the instrument yields five subscales reflecting the behavioral functions of Attention, Escape, Physical, Tangible, and Non-Social Reinforcement. Behavior checklists, such as the QABF, require little time. However, studies of their psychometrics properties suggest they should be used to offer preliminary information with additional evidence required (Matson et al., 1999; Nicholson et al., 2006; Shogren & Rojahn, 2003).

The use of a checklist was followed by a functional assessment interview conducted with caregivers (Hanley, 2012). Open-ended interviews can help gather information that may be systematically evaluated at a later stage (Slaton et al., 2017). In the interview, we asked detailed questions about the antecedents and consequences of their children's OCB to gather further detail on the functions of each behavior as identified by the QABF. The goal of this is to discover both common and unique variables that evoke or maintain OCBs. We have included the Open-Ended Functional Assessment Interview (FAI; Hanley, 2012) in Appendix A: Functional Assessment Interview to support the identification of functions.

Indirect assessments can be completed with knowledgeable informants, such as caregivers, family, and teachers. They are best completed with people who spend the most time with the individual and can be completed by people together to facilitate consensus (e.g., with both caregivers). Depending on the assessment selected, they can take as little as 10 minutes (e.g., QABF; Matson & Vollmer, 1995) and up to 90 minutes (e.g., the FAI; Hanley, 2012).

Descriptive Assessments

Descriptive assessments involve direct observation of the OCB, without any manipulation of the environmental conditions. The most common approach is an ABC (antecedent, behavior, consequence) descriptive analysis, in which you or a caregiver observe the client on multiple occasions, recording antecedent conditions, the client's behavior, and a description of the consequences of the behavior. Clinicians then review all instances of the OCB and look for relationships between the OCB and the consequences. Direct observations may be done by clinicians, teachers, and family members. Observers record when a behavior occurs, the antecedents (what happened before), the consequences (what happened after the behavior), and what their perception of the function of the behavior was in that instance. Information is collected on multiple instances to determine patterns that identify the function of the behavior, the context for the behavior, and the consequences maintaining the behavior. We have included a sample ABC form to support building on information obtained from indirect methods in Appendix B: ABC Narrative Form.

While we have used descriptive assessments to support determining function (e.g., Sheen et al., 2024), descriptive assessments have limitations in their validity (Thompson & Iwata, 2007). First, it is often difficult to capture all the relevant antecedent variables within a descriptive analysis. Second, descriptive assessments are likely to have false positives for attention, often because the target behavior cannot be ignored by people around them (Thompson & Iwata, 2007). Therefore, we often recommend omitting long descriptive assessments. Brief, open-ended observations, such as those described in the defining section may be useful for creating an observable and measurable definition, as well as identifying particular antecedent-consequence that often co-occur that could be relevant for treatment. They may also be useful when the interview does not lead to information to support further assessment (Hanley, 2012).

In our work, we observed youth behavior in contrived and naturally occurring situations at home and during therapy sessions. Caregivers also recorded videos of child behavior at home that were later analyzed by clinicians, Analysis of antecedents, consequences, and possible functions was conducted by researchers trained in applied behavior analysis (ABA).

Functional Analysis

Functional analysis involves the experimental manipulation of environmental events to test the different possible functions of the client's behavior. During a functional analysis, you observe the level of responding while systematically manipulating the environment. These analyses are the most precise, rigorous and controlled methods used in conducting a functional assessment and are the only method that allows for unambiguous demonstration of the functional relationships between behavior and the environment. Recent research includes methods for addressing low-rate and covert behavior (Hanley, 2012) and analyses that are brief (Jessel et al., 2016). However, identifying and treating automatically maintained behavior using functional analysis still presents some challenges (Hagopian et al., 2018, 2023).

Because functional analysis involves creating situations that will or are likely to provoke OCBs and because their success requires training, it is recommended that functional analyses be conducted only with the involvement of a person trained in conducting functional analyses and ABA. Moreover, functional analysis can be difficult to conduct when OCBs serve non-socially mediated automatic functions – for example, automatic positive reinforcement (seeking out pleasant sensations) and/or automatic negative reinforcement (avoiding aversive sensations) – particularly if the individual is unable to describe their internal state. Our emphasis, therefore, in this work is on indirect and descriptive methods because we believe those are the most applicable during the nine-week treatment protocol. Without manipulation, these functions cannot be empirically validated, so we refer to them as perceived functions.

Summarizing Function

The main outcome of the functional assessment process involves integrating the information into hypothesis statements about the OCBs. These statements describe the context (setting events and antecedents), the OCB, the consequences, and the function the OCB serves. You should attempt to develop a hypothesis statement for each OCB or group of OCBs that appear to serve a particular function.

Box 3.3   Examples of Summary Statements

1. When John has not had breakfast in the morning and is given a difficult math assignment, he yells and hits his desk, which results in him being sent to the principal's office by his teacher. The perceived function of the behavior is socially mediated escape from a difficult task.
2. When Alyssa has a difficult homework assignment to complete after dinner, she will claim that her hands are dirty and delay

or avoid the work by going to wash her hands for an hour or more. The perceived function of the excessive handwashing is non-socially mediated negative reinforcement (avoidance of homework).

3. Carla brings home her backpack full of garbage from school almost every day. Her mother spends time with her emptying the pack and throwing out the garbage while explaining to Carla that she should not bring home garbage from school. The perceived function of this OCB is socially mediated access to parental attention.

The goal of the functional assessment is to identify the function(s) of the OCBs. The hypothesis statement summarizes what is understood about antecedents, behavior, and consequences. From here, a multicomponent function-based intervention plan is designed to make the OCB irrelevant, ineffective, or inefficient (O'Neill et al., 2015). Function-based intervention strategies address aspects of the context, such as preventative strategies that focus on minimizing the effects of EOs and removing or altering antecedents.

Diagramming Function

When summarizing functions, you should draw a diagram that outlines the context for OCB (antecedents and setting events), the behavior, and the consequences maintaining behavior as in Figure 3.2. We have provided a sheet in Appendix C: Competing Behavior Model Form for summarizing the functional assessment process and planning function-based interventions. At the top of the page is a competing behavior model. Use this space to create a diagram that outlines the setting events, antecedents, behavior, and consequences. In a competing behavior model, you should also identify one or more alternative replacement behaviors that the child could perform to achieve the same outcome as the OCB.

Consider the example of Michael, who engaged in repetitive questioning and reassurance seeking from his mother about germs and getting sick. The functional behavior assessment consisted of administering indirect assessments (the QABF and a functional assessment interview) and conducting direct observations using an ABC checklist. Combining the results of both indirect and direct assessment, perceived functions

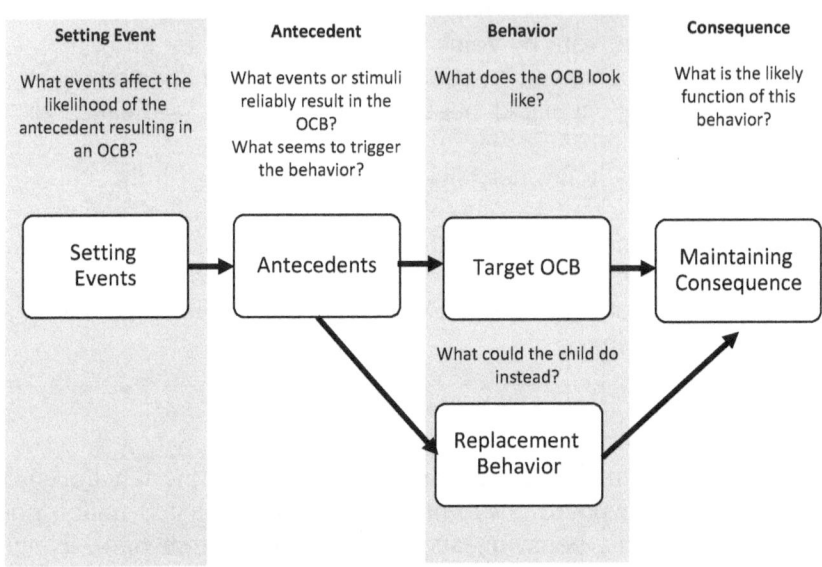

Figure 3.2 Summary diagram of function.

were escape from anxiety and access to attention. We found that Michael was likely to seek reassurance when presented with non-social or independent activities, and this behavior increased when others in the household were sick. During our treatment, Michael's sibling had a severe illness resulting in a hospital visit which was associated with a large increase in this behavior. We hypothesized the behavior was maintained by automatic negative reinforcement in the form of escape from anxiety and socially mediated positive reinforcement in the form of parental attention. Table 3.2 presents a summary diagram of Michael's functional assessment.

In Chapter 1, we discussed Camden, a 12-year-old youth who engaged in repetitive handwashing. Initially, Camden expressed fears about contamination and germs that resulted in a feeling of needing to wash his hands for long periods of time. Descriptive assessments suggested handwashing was maintained by non-socially mediated negative reinforcement. Later in treatment, we also observed enjoyment such as smiling and commentary about the feeling of the warm water, suggesting a non-socially mediated access function. That is, the sensory stimulation from the warm water acted as automatic positive reinforcement. Table 3.3 presents a summary diagram for Camden's functional assessment.

Table 3.2 Summary Diagram of Function for Michael

Establishing Operation(s)	Antecedent(s)	OCB(s)	Maintaining Consequence(s)	Function(s)
Brother was sick	Mealtime, presence of others who were sick	Repeatedly asking for reassurance	Escape from anxiety; access to parental attention	Non-socially mediated escape from anxiety; socially mediated access to parent attention

Table 3.3 Summary Diagram of Function for Camden

Establishing Operation(s)	Antecedent(s)	OCB(s)	Maintaining Consequence(s)	Function(s)
Limited use or play with water	Child is near a sink and soap	Washing hands for extended periods	Escape from anxiety; access to sensory stimulation	Non-socially-mediated escape from anxiety; Non-socially-mediated access to sensory stimulation

Function vs. Topography

A common trap is to choose an intervention procedure based on the topography of the OCB (what the behavior looks like) rather than on the function of the behavior. For example, because extended handwashing is a common obsessive-compulsive disorder (OCD) symptom, interventions that address non-socially mediated negative reinforcement functions (i.e., escape from distress) such as cognitive restructuring and exposure/response prevention (E/RP) often are selected. For behavior that is more commonly seen among the restricted and/or repetitive behaviors (RRBs) of autism, clinicians might tend to rely more heavily on traditional ABA-based interventions, such as replacing RRBs with appropriate toy play. Although each focus (CBT or ABA) might result in measurable decreases in the OCB in some situations, the intervention is likely to be ineffective if the clinician is not addressing all functions of the behavior or potentially inadvertently reinforcing the behavior. Further, the same behavior topography can serve different functions for different individuals. For example, throughout our work, we have addressed the OCB of sitting in the same seat. In some instances, perceived functions included access to parental attention, and in other instances, children clearly articulated distress related to fears of contamination. Knowing the function of the OCB and linking the function to intervention increases the likelihood of choosing an effective approach.

Summary of the Functional Assessment Process

The main outcomes of a functional assessment are (1) a clear description of the OCB including precursor behavior; (2) an identification of the immediate antecedents that predict or trigger OCB; (3) identification of general or more distal setting events that influence the likelihood of OCB by making it more or less sensitive to antecedent and consequences; (4) identification of the consequences that maintain OCB and potential function it may serve; and (5) development of a summary chart that describes the relationship between OCB, the context (antecedents and setting events), and their perceived function (maintaining consequences).

Function-Based Interventions

Replacement Behavior and Functional Communication Training

Teaching new skills is the most effective approach for creating lasting change in OCB, and knowing the function of the behavior allows you to select skills that will serve the same function as the behavior and serve as a replacement for the OCB. One such approach is called functional communication training (FCT; Carr & Durand, 1985). It is an evidence-based intervention used to reduce interfering behavior or less clear communication forms by teaching alternative communication strategies. Alternative communication strategies can include vocal requests, gestures, or communication devices. Using differential reinforcement, the child is taught a replacement response that serves the same function or results in the same reinforcement that has been identified as maintaining the interfering behavior. To implement FCT, first a functional assessment is completed to identify the function of the behavior, then a simple replacement response is identified and taught to the child. Finally, the replacement response is strengthened by providing access to the same reinforcer(s) that maintained the interfering behavior. To maximize the effectiveness of FCT, the replacement communication response should be efficient and easy to do (preferably have

Table 3.4 Examples of Replacement Behaviors That Serve the Same Function

Function of Behavior	Topography	Potential Replacement
Socially mediated access to parental attention	Asking for reassurance about scars or marks on their body	Teach them how to initiate conversations about preferred topics
Non-socially mediated escape from anxiety	Sitting in the same seat at the dinner table	Teach relaxation and coping techniques; reinforce sitting in different locations.
Socially mediated escape from difficult situations	Avoiding competitive games, elopement	Teach how to ask for help when games are difficult or unclear; reinforce participation

less energy expenditure than the interfering behavior), reliably access reinforcement, and obtain as much, if not more, of the reinforcer maintaining interfering behavior.

Table 3.4 provides some examples of matching replacement behaviors that serve the same function as the OCB.

For example, a functional assessment might identify that access to caregiver attention likely maintains an OCB, FCT could involve teaching a child how to initiate a conversation to access social attention and increased involvement with a caregiver. Similarly, a child who engages in an OCB to avoid difficult tasks can be taught to request a break using picture card or simple phrases like, "Break, please." When the child uses the card or phrase, they are given a set time (e.g., five minutes) away from the task. Children can also be taught to request help, rather than a break in contexts where the behavior serves as escape from difficult tasks function. Then assistance to make the task easier can be provided promptly when the replacement response is demonstrated. Children can also be taught to request access to items or activities to replace OCBs that serve socially mediated access functions (e.g., "more, please"). When designing replacement responses, therapists should consider responses that are likely to be effective in multiple contexts (e.g., something a novel conversation partner would recognize) and that can be acquired quickly or that are already in the child's repertoire (Tiger et al., 2008).

Selecting Intervention Strategies

Function-based intervention plans are often multicomponent, and while identifying a functional replacement behavior is a key aspect of a function-based intervention plan, there are other components of the environment where the clinician can intervene that will reduce the likelihood of the OCB and increase the likelihood of replacement behavior. To do this, clinicians can implement strategies that act on both the antecedents and the consequences present. Table 3.5 provides various ways that clinicians reduce the likelihood of an OCB occurring and increase the likelihood of a functional replacement occurring.

Consider strategies that might eliminate or reduce the effects of **EOs or setting events**. Changes in these can make OCBs irrelevant. For example, if deprivation of parental interaction serves as an EO for repetitive question-asking before bedtime, scheduling 30 minutes of high-quality activities with a parent before the bedtime routine can reduce the EO for parental attention as a reinforcer and result in decreased question-asking.

Changes in immediate **antecedent** events can also reduce the likelihood of OCBs. For example, consider how changes in the level of assistance, how instructions are delivered, the length and difficulty of the task, etc., might reduce the aversiveness of tasks, serving to decrease the value of escape as a reinforcer.

Table 3.5 Function-Based Strategies

Setting Event Strategies	Antecedent Strategies	Behavior Strategies	Consequence Strategies
Prevent setting events from occurring (e.g., ensure adequate sleep, resolve medication issues) Neutralize setting events (e.g., provide a nap, provide a break after a conflict)	Offer choices Modify antecedents (e.g., make tasks less difficult, shorter) Prompt replacement behavior before OCB occurs Provide preferred items as a distractor (e.g., watching a tablet during a dentist appointment) Provide non-contingent access to reinforcer (e.g., increased parental attention)	Teach communicative behaviors that can replace the OCB and can serve the same function using modeling, prompting, and reinforcement (e.g., teach the child to ask for a break or recruit attention) Build related skills (e.g., teach initiation and conversation skills) Teach independent leisure and play skills that access same sensory reinforcement as OCB (e.g., water play) Teach coping strategies for emotional regulation	Provide reinforcement for replacement behavior Minimize reinforcement for OCB Redirect to appropriate behavior or coping strategies

Teaching Replacement Behavior

In addition to identifying function-based strategies and replacement behavior, clinicians need to identify strategies for teaching and promoting replacement behavior. Just knowing how to perform a replacement behavior does not mean the child will be able to perform that skill in the desired context. For example, a child may know how to ask for help in some contexts (at school) but not in others (with caregivers). It is also possible that the child performs the OCB because it is more effective than other behaviors; it is currently functional. Strategies should then also focus on replacement responses that are more efficient and effective than OCBs. For example, a child may know how to initiate a conversation about preferred topics, which their family members ignore. When the child begins talking about death and dying, the family then responds to them. In this instance, the OCB is more efficient at obtaining family members' attention. Introducing a means to engage with family members and coaching family members to respond to bids for attention will result in that pathway being selected more often than talking about death and dying (which should be redirected to other topics).

If the child needs to be taught a replacement behavior, there are a multitude of behavioral intervention strategies for doing so. Instruction should focus on how to perform the behavior as well as when those behaviors are appropriate. Behavioral skills training (see Chapter 1 for more detail) can be used to teach replacement behavior. Some children might require more intensive instructional procedures that involve breaking the skill into smaller steps (begin with "break" before, "Can I have a break, please?"), providing visual aids, models, and prompts to increase the likelihood of performing the behavior, correcting or providing feedback on errors (or ignoring them if appropriate), and providing praise and reinforcement for responses that meet the goal criteria.

Finally, clinicians need to consider how **consequences** can be altered to make the replacement behavior pathway more likely. If the OCB produces a powerful reinforcer, clinicians can increase the value of the reinforcer associated with engaging in replacement responses and decrease the value of the reinforcer associated with the OCB. For example, for a response maintained by access to adult attention, reducing the amount of attention provided for the OCB and providing access to high-quality attention contingent on the replacement response.

Table 3.6 provides examples of strategies to address setting events, antecedents and consequences as well as potential replacement behaviors that address the function of behavior. The strategies listed in Table 3.6 are not meant to be exhaustive, but rather potential examples.

Table 3.6 Function-Based Strategies

Escaping or Avoiding Tasks or Environments

Strategy	Examples
Adjust the difficulty and length of the task	Provide easier tasks Break down task into smaller steps Decrease expectations Shorten the task Provide frequent breaks
Offer choice	Child can choose: • Which tasks to complete • The order • What materials • Where to complete the task • When to complete the task • With whom to complete the task • Reinforcer earned for task completion
Incorporate child interests	Include the child's interests in the activity (e.g., addition and subtraction with favorite characters)
Modify the way the child completes the task	Type responses rather than write them
Use behavioral momentum	Provide easy tasks before more difficult tasks
Modify the instructions	Present one instruction at a time Talk slower Use preferred mode (e.g., typed, oral, written, visuals) Use a different tone of voice (e.g., excited) First-then instructions (e.g., "First finish your homework, then you can play video games")
Teach a replacement for OCB	Provide help based on a replacement behavior (e.g., asking for help). Allow a break from instruction based on a replacement behavior (e.g., asking for a break)
Schedules	Provide breaks from activity based on a time-schedule Visual schedules using first-then (less preferred activities alternating with preferred activities)

(Continued)

Table 3.6 (Continued)

Access Tangible or Activities

Strategy	Examples
Schedule a transitional activity	Avoid transitions for more to less preferred activities when possible
	Allow access to a moderately preferred activity in between transitions from highly preferred to less preferred activities
Increase access	Put highly preferred items in easy-to-access places
	Make them more frequently accessible
	Provide the activity on a time-based schedule
Teach a replacement for OCB	Provide the preferred item or activity when the child performs a replacement behavior (e.g., asking for the item)

Access Attention

Strategy	Examples
Schedule attention	Have target person (adult, peer) provide attention and engage with child in their preferred activities on a time based or periodic schedule
	Have an adult work with a child
	Have a peer work with the child
	Create a buddy system
Provide a replacement activity	When person is occupied and unable to provide attention, give the child a preferred activity
Teach a replacement for OCB	Provide attention when the child performs a replacement behavior (e.g., starting a conversation)

Escape from Social Situations

Strategy	Examples
Intersperse activities	Create schedules where there is time away from a group or person
	Embed independent work or place

(Continued)

Table 3.6 (Continued)

Escape from Social Situations

Strategy	Examples
Alter proximity	Change seating arrangements at dinner or in car to separate less preferred people or attention
Teach the child strategies that allow them to control the environment	Putting headphones on in the car or bus to minimize noise and attention from others
Teach a replacement for OCB	Remove attention when the child performs a replacement behavior (e.g., says I need to be alone)

Access Sensory Stimulation

Strategy	Examples
Provide an alternative activity	Offer items or activities that match the type of sensation that OCB creates (e.g., water play in place of handwashing)
Enrich the environment	Provide environment with lots of interesting activities and objects
Teach the child strategies that allow them to control the environment	How to use laptops, tablets, and/or phones to watch videos, listen to music, and play video games How to control lighting

Escape from Sensory Stimulation

Strategy	Examples
Provide an alternative activity	Noise cancelling headphones or earbuds to listen to preferred music Quiet room
Enrich the environment	Provide an environment with preferred forms of sensory stimulation
Teach the child strategies that allow them to control the environment	How to turn off lighting How to turn on and off fans How to control TV volume

The Role of Skill Building

Teaching skills is the most effective strategy for creating lasting change in behavior. Knowing the perceived function of OCB allows us to select skills that can serve the same function as the behavior and work as a replacement. As a therapist, it is important to ask what the child will be doing now that they are not doing the OCB. Further, sometimes

OCBs arise from, or overlap with skill deficits. For example, challenges with daily living and self-care routines might interact with extended toothbrushing or washing routines. Difficulty initiating conversations with others might interact with repetitive questions or reassurance seeking. In cases where skill deficits overlap with OCBs, it can be beneficial to incorporate systematic instructional procedures. This might involve task analyses to break skills down into parts, providing multiple teaching opportunities, including modeling and prompting to prevent errors, systematically fading support, praising and providing reinforcement for accurate responses and providing corrective feedback for errors.

As discussed earlier, Michael engaged in repetitive questioning and reassurance seeking from his mother about germs and getting sick. After completing the FBA, we hypothesized the OCB was maintained by automatic negative reinforcement in the form of escape from anxiety and socially mediated positive reinforcement in the form of parental attention. Table 3.7 presents a competing behavior model for Michael. A replacement behavior for Michael was identified that produced the same consequence as the OCB. To address the access to parental attention function, Michael was taught ways to initiate conversations about his interests (e.g., building things) with behavioral skills training including roleplaying some "go-to" conversation starters. Starting a conversation about his interests was a suitable replacement as it would also produce parental attention. Caregivers were also coached to be active participants in conversations about his interests.

Table 3.7 Competing Behavior Model and Strategies for Michael

Establishing Operation(s)	Antecedent(s)	OCB(s)	Maintaining Consequence(s)	Function(s)
Brother was sick	Mealtime, presence of others who were sick	Asking for reassurance	Access to parental attention Escape from anxiety	Socially mediated access to parent attention Non-socially mediated escape from anxiety
		Replacement Behavior Talking about interests		

(Continued)

Table 3.7 (Continued)

Setting Event/EO Strategies	Antecedent Strategies	Teaching Strategies	Consequence Strategies
Exposure and response prevention	Remind Michael that he can start a conversation about his favorite things Remind Michael to use his coping strategies	Behavioral skills training to teach initiating conversations about his favorite things Behavioral skills training to teach self-talk and coping strategies (breathing, muscle relaxation)	Provide praise and continued conversation when talking about topics other than germs when someone is sick Reduce attention to questions about germs and redirect to other topics Provide praise for using coping strategies

To address the escape from anxiety function, we engaged Michael in exposure and response prevention, including role-playing the exposure activities. The therapist used simplified cognitive restructuring, including challenging that all germs were bad and exposure to some might support a healthy body (or immune system). Michael and the therapist generated self-talk specific to the OCB (e.g., "It's OK, some germs are good") and externalizing statements (e.g., bug off OCB) as cognitive strategies. We used behavioral skills training to teach Michael diaphragmatic breathing and progressive muscle relaxation, and he also talked about his favorite things as coping strategies. Parents were encouraged to provide praise when they saw Michael engaging in breathing or muscle relaxation exercises and provide less attention to questions about germs.

For Camden, intervention primarily focused on eliminating EOs (Table 3.8). We addressed the non-socially mediated negative reinforcement function with exposure and response prevention to reduce the EO of distress, gradually decreasing the duration of handwashing. Similar to Michael, we used cognitive restructuring to decrease the association between germs and sickness. We used behavioral skills training to teach self-talk statements specific to the OCB (e.g., "Some germs are good for you" and "I can wash for two minutes!") and behavioral strategies including taking deep breaths. Camden identified that washing hands produced non-socially mediated reinforcement; they liked the feeling

Table 3.8 Competing Behavior Model and Function-Based Strategies for Camden

Establishing Operation(s)	Antecedent(s)	OCB(s)	Maintaining Consequence(s)	Function(s)
Limited use or play with water	Child is near a sink and soap	Washing hands	Access to sensory stimulation Escape from anxiety	Non-socially-mediated access to sensory stimulation Non-socially-mediated escape from anxiety
		Replacement Behavior Using fountain ↗		

Setting Event/EO Strategies	Antecedent Strategies	Teaching Strategies	Consequence Strategies
Provide ongoing access to water fountain Exposure and response prevention	Remind Camden they can use the fountain	Behavioral skills training to teach self-talk and coping strategies (breathing)	None

of the warm water on their hands during handwashing. We identified a functional replacement behavior that produced a similar sensation involving accessing warm water from a small indoor fountain, that the family already had present in the home. By providing free access to the fountain, we aimed to decrease the establishing operation for handwashing by providing an alternative that would satisfy the potential regulatory need. Since the alternative behavior could potentially become a compulsion, therapists also monitored the level of fountain use to ensure it did not increase to interfering levels.

Summarizing Function-Based Interventions for Caregivers

Once you have completed the competing behavior model worksheet (Appendix X) for planning the function-based intervention for yourself, you will need to train caregivers in the implementation. Caregiver training to complete function-based interventions begins in Session 3 and during the caregiver modules each week, and detailed instructions for conducting these are within each session. In preparation for these sessions, you will need to outline the function-based intervention plan for caregivers. We have provided a sheet in Appendix D (FBAI Summary Form) that you can use to create a handout, and a sample complete one can be found in Session 2. Each week you will list the target OCB, next to each OCB you will list the hypothesized function of the OCB (e.g., access to caregiver attention), and finally you will list strategies to reduce the OCB. You can continue to add OCBs as treatment progresses. List all the functions for caregivers (e.g., escape from anxiety and access to attention). You can simplify the language you use to report functions by using access and escape followed by the hypothesized reinforcer (e.g., escape from math homework). For escape from anxiety functions, refer caregivers to the cognitive and behavioral skills training that occurs in session, identifying strategies that the child selected or preferred.

References

American Psychiatric Association. (2022). *Diagnostic and statistical manual of mental disorders* (5th ed., text rev.). https://doi.org/10.1176/appi.books.9780890425787

Carr, E. G., & Durand, V. M. (1985). Reducing behavior problems through functional communication training. *Journal of Applied Behavior Analysis*, *18*(2), 111–126. https://doi.org/10.1901/jaba.1985.18-111

Cooper, J. O., Heron, T. E., & Heward, W. L. (2019). *Applied behavior analysis* (3rd ed.). Pearson Education, Inc.

Guertin, E. L., Vause, T., Thomson, K. M., Frijters, J. C., & Feldman, M. A. (2022). Obsessive–compulsive behaviors in autism spectrum disorder: Behavior analytic conceptual frameworks. *Behavior Analysis: Research and Practice*, *22*(1), 81–99. https://doi.org/10.1037/bar0000236

Hagopian, L. P., Falligant, J. M., Frank-Crawford, M. A., Yenokyan, G., Piersma, D. E., & Kaur, J. (2023). Simplified methods for identifying subtypes of automatically maintained self-injury. *Journal of Applied Behavior Analysis*, *56*(3), 575–592. https://doi.org/10.1002/JABA.1005

Hagopian, L. P., Rooker, G. W., & Yenokyan, G. (2018). Identifying predictive behavioral markers: A demonstration using automatically reinforced self-injurious behavior. *Journal of Applied Behavior Analysis*, *51*(3), 443–465. https://doi.org/10.1002/JABA.477

Hanley, G. P. (2012). Functional assessment of problem behavior: Dispelling myths, overcoming implementation obstacles, and developing new lore. *Behavior Analysis in Practice*, *5*(1), 54. https://doi.org/10.1007/BF03391818

Hanley, G. P., Jin, C. S., Vanselow, N. R., & Hanratty, L. A. (2014). Producing meaningful improvements in problem behavior of children with autism via synthesized analyses and treatments. *Journal of Applied Behavior Analysis*, *47*(1), 16–36. https://doi.org/10.1002/jaba.106

Jessel, J., Hanley, G. P., & Ghaemmaghami, M. (2016). Interview-informed synthesized contingency analyses: Thirty replications and reanalysis. *Journal of Applied Behavior Analysis*, *49*(3), 576–595. https://doi.org/10.1002/JABA.316

Love, J. R., Carr, J. E., & Leblanc, L. A. (2009). Functional assessment of problem behavior in children with autism spectrum disorders: A summary of 32 outpatient cases. *Journal of Autism and Developmental Disorders*, *39*(2), 363–372. https://doi.org/10.1007/s10803-008-0633-z

Lynch, C. L. (2019, March 28). Invisible abuse: ABA and the things only autistic people can see. *The Aspergan*. 30. https://neuroclastic.com/invisible-abuse-aba-and-the-things-only-autistic-people-can-see/

Martin, G., & Pear, J. (2024). Behavior modification: What it is and how to do it, 12th edition. In *Behavior modification: What it is and how to do it* (12th ed.). https://doi.org/10.4324/9781003276722

Matson, J. L., Bamburg, J. W., Cherry, K. E., & Paclawskyj, T. R. (1999). A validity study on the questions about behavioral function (QABF) scale: Predicting treatment success for self-injury, aggression, and stereotypies. *Research in Developmental Disabilities, 20*(2), 163–175. https://doi.org/10.1016/S0891-4222(98)00039-0

Matson, J. L., & Vollmer, T. R. (1995). *User's guide: Questions about behavioral function (QABF)*. Scientific Publishers, Inc.

Michael, J. (1993). Establishing operations. *The Behavior Analyst, 16*(2), 191–206. https://doi.org/10.1007/BF03392623

Mowrer, O. H. (1951). Two-factor learning theory: Summary and comment. *Psychological Review, 58*(5), 350–354. https://doi.org/10.1037/H0058956

Nicholson, J., Konstantinidi, E., & Furniss, F. (2006). On some psychometric properties of the questions about behavioral function (QABF) scale. *Research in Developmental Disabilities, 27*(3), 337–352. https://doi.org/10.1016/J.RIDD.2005.04.001

O'Neill, R. E., Albin, R. W., Storey, K., Horner, R. H., & Sprague, J. R. (2015). *Functional assessment and program development for problem behavior: A practical handbook* (3rd ed.). Cengage Learning.

Paclawskyj, T. R., Matson, J. L., Rush, K. S., Smalls, Y., & Vollmer, T. R. (2000). Questions about behavioral function (QABF): A behavioral checklist for functional assessment of aberrant behavior. *Research in Developmental Disabilities, 21*(3), 223–229. https://doi.org/10.1016/S0891-4222(00)00036-6

Reese, R. M., Richman, D. M., Zarcone, J., & Zarcone, T. (2003). Individualizing functional assessments for children with Autism. *Focus on Autism and Other Developmental Disabilities, 18*(2), 89–94. https://doi.org/10.1177/108835760301800202

Rodriguez, N. M., Thompson, R. H., Schlichenmeyer, K., & Stocco, C. S. (2012). Functional analysis and treatment of arranging and ordering by individuals with autism spectrum disorder. *Journal of Applied Behavior Analysis, 45*(1), 1–22. https://doi.org/10.1901/jaba.2012.45-1

Sheen, H., Vause, T., Neil, N., Anderson, B. M., & Feldman, M. A. (2024). Functional analysis and treatment of hoarding in a child with autism spectrum disorder. *Behavior Analysis in Practice*. Advance online publication. https://doi.org/10.1007/s40617-024-00967-5

Shogren, K. A., & Rojahn, J. (2003). Convergent reliability and validity of the questions about behavioral function and the motivation assessment scale: A replication study. *Journal of Developmental and Physical Disabilities, 15*(4), 367–375. https://doi.org/10.1023/A:1026314316977/METRICS

Slaton, J. D., & Hanley, G. P. (2018). Nature and scope of synthesis in functional analysis and treatment of problem behavior. *Journal of Applied Behavior Analysis, 51*(4), 943–973. https://doi.org/10.1002/JABA.498

Slaton, J. D., Hanley, G. P., & Raftery, K. J. (2017). Interview-informed functional analyses: A comparison of synthesized and isolated components. *Journal of Applied Behavior Analysis, 50*(2), 252–277. https://doi.org/10.1002/JABA.384

Thompson, R. H., & Iwata, B. A. (2007). A comparison of outcomes from descriptive and functional analyses of problem behavior. *Journal of Applied Behavior Analysis, 40*(2), 333–338. https://doi.org/10.1901/jaba.2007.56-06

Tiger, J. H., Hanley, G. P., & Bruzek, J. (2008). Functional communication training: A review and practical guide. *Behavior Analysis in Practice, 1*(1), 16. https://doi.org/10.1007/BF03391716

Vause, T., Neil, N., Jaksic, H., Jackiewicz, G., & Feldman, M. (2017). Preliminary randomized trial of function-based cognitive-behavioral therapy to treat obsessive compulsive behavior in children with autism spectrum disorder. *Focus on Autism and Other Developmental Disabilities, 32*(3), 218–228. https://doi.org/10.1177/1088357615588517

Appendix A

Functional Assessment Interview

Open-Ended Functional Assessment Interview

Developed by Gregory P. Hanley, Ph.D., BCBA-D
(Developed August 2002; Revised: August 2009 and February 2022)

Date of Interview: _____
Child/Client: _____
Respondent: _____
Respondent's relation to child/client: _____
Interviewer: _____

RELEVANT BACKGROUND INFORMATION

1. His/her date of birth and current age: ____-_____-_____ ____yrs ____mos Male/Female
2. Describe his/her language abilities.
3. Describe his/her play skills and preferred toys or leisure activities.
4. What else does he/she prefer?

QUESTIONS TO INFORM THE DESIGN OF A FUNCTIONAL ANALYSIS

To develop objective definitions of observable problem behaviors:
5. What are the problem behaviors? What do they look like?

To determine which problem behavior(s) will be targeted in the functional analysis:
6. What is the single-most concerning problem behavior?
7. What are the top 3 most concerning problem behaviors? Are there other behaviors of concern?

To determine the precautions required when conducting the functional analysis:
8. Describe the range of intensities of the problem behaviors and the extent to which he/she or others may be hurt or injured from the problem behavior.

To assist in identifying precursors to or behavioral indicators of dangerous problem behaviors that may be targeted in the functional analysis instead of more dangerous problem behaviors:

9. Do the different types of problem behavior tend to occur in bursts or clusters and/or does any type of problem behavior typically precede another type of problem behavior (e.g., yells preceding hits)? Are there behaviors that seem to indicate that severe problem behavior is about to occur?

To determine the antecedent conditions that may be incorporated into the functional analysis test conditions:

10. Under what conditions or situations are the problem behaviors most likely to occur?
11. Do the problem behaviors reliably occur during any particular activities?
12. What seems to trigger the problem behavior?
13. Does problem behavior occur when you break routines or interrupt activities? If so, describe.
14. Does the problem behavior occur when it appears that he/she won't get his/her way? If so, describe the things that the child often attempts to control.

To determine the test condition(s) that should be conducted and the specific type(s) of consequences that may be incorporated into the test condition(s):

15. How do you and others react or respond to the problem behavior?
16. What do you and others do to calm him/her down once he/she engaged in the problem behavior?
17. What do you and others do to distract him/her from engaging in the problem behavior?

In addition to the given information, to assist in developing a hunch as to why problem behavior is occurring and to assist in determining the test condition(s) to be conducted:

18. What do you think he/she is trying to communicate with his/her problem behavior, if anything?
19. Do you think this problem behavior is a form of self-stimulation? If so, what gives you that impression?
20. Why do you think he/she is engaging in the problem behavior?

To ensure that the analytic context is properly designed for developing the most important skill branches.

Besides communication, toleration, and cooperation:

21. What skills would make this child/client's life better/more joyful?
22. What are the three most useful things the child/client could be taught to do?
23. What skills, if this child/client had them, would make your life or the lives of other close caregivers better?

Appendix B

ABC Narrative Form

Client Name:_____ Observer:_____

Date and Time	Antecedent Events	Behavior	Consequent Events
	(Describe what happened immediately prior to the behavior.)	(Describe what the student did in objective, observable terms.)	(Describe what happened immediately following the behavior.)

The following are some examples of possible Antecedents, Behaviors and Consequences.

Please indicate the number in the columns above and make notes about what you saw.

Possible Antecedents

1. Task presentation
2. Difficult task/activity
3. Others' comments
4. Activity change
5. Asked to wait
6. Activity denied
7. Other: _____
_____
_____

Behavior

_____

Possible Consequences

1. Task termination
2. Activity change
3. Neg. adult attention
4. Neg. peer attention
5. Pos. adult attention
6. Pos. peer attention
7. Other: _____
_____

Appendix C

Competing Behavior Model Form

Name: _____ Date:_____ OCB:_____

What events affect the likelihood of the antecedent resulting in an OCB?	What events or stimuli reliably result in the OCB? What seems to trigger the behavior?	What does the OCB look like?		What is the likely function of this behavior?
Establishing Operation(s)	**Antecedent(s)**	**OCB(s)**	**Maintaining Consequence(s)**	**Function(s)**

Replacement Behavior

Establishing Operation Strategies	**Antecedent Strategies**	**Teaching Strategies**	**Consequence Strategies**

Appendix D

Functional Behavior Assessment and Interview (FBAI) Summary Form

OCB(s) *Compulsion/Obsession*	Likely Function(s) *Why the OCB happens*	Function-based Intervention(s) *How to reduce the OCB(s)* **Implement During* *Exposure or After Gradual* *Exposure Step*
1.	1.	1.
2.	2.	2.
3.	3.	3.
4.	4.	4.
5.	5.	5.

Chapter 4

Embedded Social Skills Curriculum for Children With Autism

Introduction

Social skills are an essential component of child development. From an early age, neurotypical children seek out, initiate, and sustain social interactions with other people, such as their caregivers, siblings, and peers. In doing so, they learn critical skills, such as pre-verbal communication (e.g., eye contact, joint attention, gestures) and parallel play. As children are exposed to more social opportunities over time, these skill repertoires increase in complexity – early communication skills develop into conversational skills, and parallel play develops into cooperative play. With continued practice, complex social relationships are formed, which foster positive psychosocial outcomes and belonging.

Social Skills and Autism

Children with autism often have difficulties with social interaction and communication. One of the diagnostic criteria for autism is persistent challenges in social communication, such as difficulties with social-emotional reciprocity, nonverbal communication, and developing, maintaining, and understanding relationships (American Psychological Association [APA], 2022).

Furthermore, children with autism often engage in restrictive, repetitive behaviors, interests, and activities (APA, 2022). In this manual, we describe our functional behavior-based CBT (Fb-CBT) that tackles a large subset of higher-order repetitive behaviors (or obsessive-compulsive behaviors [OCBs]) which are commonly linked to a variety of less favorable outcomes, including decreased learning opportunities (Boyd et al., 2012, 2013), social interactions (Guertin et al., 2019), and a negative impact on quality of life (Vause et al., 2020). These behaviors often lead to increased distress (Vause et al., 2020), bullying (Zablotsky et al., 2013), and caregiver stress (Harrop et al., 2016). Typically, these

DOI: 10.4324/9781003410126-4

characteristics are present in early childhood and can interfere with developing critical social skills (Guertin et al., 2019).

That said, it is important to recognize that autism is a spectrum, meaning the presentation and severity of these characteristics can vary significantly. As such, goal selection and the teaching approach must be individualized to meet each child's unique learning needs.

Neurodiversity-Affirming Social Skills Training

Individuals with autism and related developmental disabilities communicate differently than their neurotypical counterparts. Even if they are fully verbal and can understand receptive instructions at their age level, the ways they interact with others may differ subtly. For example, autistic individuals may speak with a different prosody, rhythm, or volume than non-autistic individuals (Cummins et al., 2020; Howard & Sedgewick, 2021; Patel et al., 2023). They may include scripts (e.g., phrases borrowed from popular media) in their conversations. They may also process conversations at a slower or faster speed than others. This does not mean that these ways of socializing are "wrong" or "less than"; they are simply different.

In general, **neurodiversity-affirming teaching approaches** are ones that "appreciate the preferences, interaction styles and communication priorities of neurodivergent individuals, and places the same value on these as the preferences, interaction styles and communication priorities of neurotypical individuals" (Lawrence, 2023, para. 7).

Wise (2023) developed a hierarchy of core principles for implementing neurodiversity-affirming practices, which includes such strategies as honoring all forms of communication (not just vocal speech), individualizing strategies and the environment to meet each individual's unique needs best, and fostering an individual's ability to use their "voice" by promoting the development of self-advocacy skills (e.g., teaching an individual how to communicate when they do or do not want to participate in an activity). The entire hierarchy of core principles can be found in Figure 4.1.

Neurodiversity-affirming social skills training is a way of teaching meaningful social skills to neurodiverse individuals in a manner that affirms their lived experience, builds on their strengths, and includes them in goal setting (Mathur et al., 2024). Clinicians can incorporate neurodiversity-affirming goal setting into their social skills training by considering what is necessary for the child to learn *and* what the child *wants* to learn. Our manual emphasizes considering child voice, child initiation, and individual preferences. Considerations for teaching social skills to children with autism have been summarized in Table 4.1.

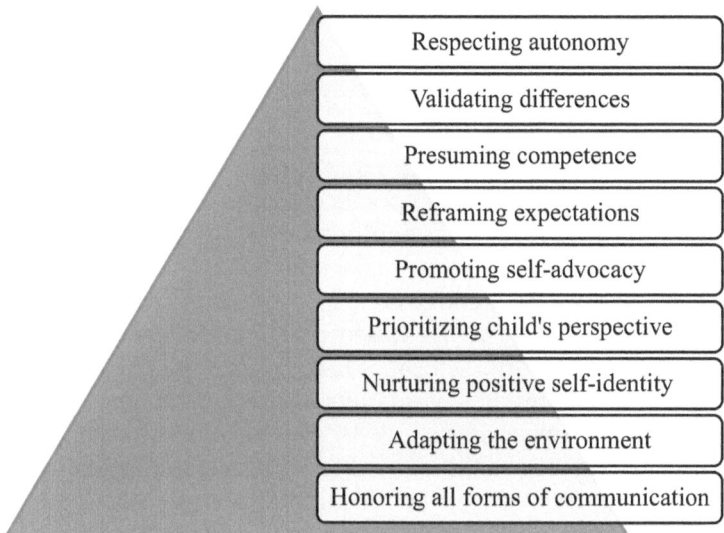

Figure 4.1 Core principles of neurodiversity-affirming practice (adapted from Wise, 2023).

Table 4.1 Considerations for Teaching Social Skills to Children With Autism

	Social skill is not necessary, adaptive, or socially meaningful.	Social skill is necessary, adaptive, or socially meaningful.
Child is interested in learning the social skill.	If time permits, teach these social skills, but consider embedding additional important skills into the teaching session (e.g., imitation).	Prioritize teaching these social skills.
Child is not interested in learning the social skill.	Do not teach these social skills.	Teach these social skills; however, embed the child's interests into the activity (e.g., use the child's favorite characters to give the instructions), provide ample reinforcement for the child's engagement in learning, and incorporate choice and child voice as often as possible.

Evidence-Based Social Skills Interventions

Several intervention components have been successful in teaching social skills to children with autism (e.g., Bauminger, 2007; Beaumont & Sofronoff, 2008; Frankel et al., 2010). It is best practice for social skills interventions to (a) use techniques that address existing skill deficits via a curriculum hierarchy, (b) incorporate activities that capture the unique motivations of each child, (c) minimize OCB and maladaptive cognitions, and (d) include a caregiver coaching component.

First, a **curriculum hierarchy** or a progression from least to most complex skills is an evidence-based practice for teaching new skills (Bauminger, 2007; Martin & Pear, 2024). For example, teaching a child to approach a communicative partner is a communication skill often taught prior to conversational skills. This ensures the child has the necessary prerequisite skills needed to be successful in learning more advanced skills and reduces their likelihood of frustration (Noell et al., 2014). Furthermore, additional support and/or adaptations, such as gestures, modeling, or visual cues, may be needed in the initial teaching stages to help the child successfully learn the skill. As the child progresses, this support can be gradually reduced or eliminated so the child learns to perform the skill with as much independence as possible. **Motivation** also plays a critical role in learning. When motivation has been established before learning, a child is more likely to engage in the skills being taught (Martin & Pear, 2024). For example, when a child is motivated to obtain a checkmark (associated with a backup reinforcer) on our Stepping It Up Completing My Exposures worksheet, which is obtained by engaging in specific coping strategies, they will be more likely to use these coping strategies than if they were indifferent to obtaining a checkmark. In addition to addressing skill deficits, previous studies have focused on **reducing OCBs**, maladaptive cognitions, and other anxiety-related behaviors that can interfere with the development of social skills (Bauminger, 2002; Wood et al., 2010). Last, **caregiver involvement** contributes to the long-term maintenance of treatment gains when addressing OCBs (Barrett, 1998; Cobham et al., 1998; Manassis et al., 2014).

Social Skills Components Included in Our Functional Behavior-Based Cognitive Behavioral Therapy

Fb-CBT is a comprehensive curriculum that primarily focuses on reducing OCBs while progressively fostering social-communicative skills. To teach social-communication skills, we have adopted best practices in our curriculum. Specifically, our Fb-CBT curriculum includes an overview of each of the exercises practiced across the nine sessions offered in our *I Believe in ME, not OCB!* treatment manual. For each exercise, the key objective, the targeted social skills, and the difficulty level of the respective social skills are also highlighted.

Our Fb-CBT curriculum teaches foundational skills before progressing to more complex skills – a structure that is consistent across other hierarchy-based curriculum tools, such as *The Assessment of Basic Language and Learning Skills-Revised* (Partington, 2006), *Verbal Behavior Milestones Assessment and Placement Program* (Sundberg, 2008), and *Social Skills Solutions* (Krempa & McKinnon, 2002). We have divided the exercises into three difficulty levels – beginner, intermediate, and advanced (see Table 4.2 for more detail). With **beginner** activities, children and youth typically require support initiating and sustaining the exercise and social interaction. These exercises require simple social interactions, such as attending to others, parallel play, and early problem-solving. With **intermediate** activities, children typically require support either initiating or sustaining the exercise or social interaction. These exercises require more complex social interactions, such as multiple or sustained responses, and understanding the intended purpose of various social interactions. With **advanced** activities, children require

Beginner

- Children require support initiating and sustaining the activity or social interaction.
- Exercise requires simple social interactions.
- Example: Following simple instructions while sitting in a group.

Intermediate

- Children may require support initiating and/or sustaining the activity or social interaction.
- Exercise requires more complex social interactions.
- Example: Engaging in a simple relay race while a peer does the same.

Advanced

- Children require minimal or no support initiating or sustaining the activity or social interaction.
- Exercise requires complex social interactions.
- Example: Engaging in a cooperative relay race with a peer.

Figure 4.2 Level of difficulty for our social skills activities.

minimal support initiating and sustaining the exercise and/or social interaction. These exercises require self-management skills, understanding social rules, and generalizing social skills to novel activities.

The exercises are designed to be fun, engaging, and suitable for this target age group (7 to 13 years). They are also **ecologically valid**, meaning the exercises and social skills are taught in a way the child's same-age peers may have also learned them. Additional practice opportunities are included to ensure foundational skills have been established.

Box 4.1   Teaching Social Skills in Individual Therapy Sessions

Teaching social skills may come naturally when leading therapy sessions of two or more children; however, it should still be prioritized even during one-on-one therapy. The social skills activities included in *I Believe in Me, Not OCB!* can be adapted for use in individual therapy sessions. Where applicable, we have included possible modifications for each activity; however, we encourage you to be creative and modify the activities to meet the child's unique needs and interests!

I Believe in Me, Not OCB! Social Skills Activities

Session Rules

Session rules (Session 1, Children's Workbook) establish session expectations. Group rules are a **beginner** skill that helps children build communication skills, such as attending to others and following simple instructions; group skills, such as waiting a turn and remaining seated in a group; and self-regulation, such as tolerating new rules and expectations.

Instructions: Ask each child to flip to the page in their workbook that has a set of "session rules" to follow. These should be reviewed for both group and individual therapy. Explain why we need rules and read each rule (or have children read the rules aloud). Use role-playing with the visuals in the workbook to provide a visual demonstration of each rule. If children are willing, have them read the rules aloud, and participate in role-playing. For example, you may read the rule "keep your hands and feet to yourselves and respect the personal space of others," and have the members do an exercise where they put their arms out and turn around in a circle. You can indicate that this is how much space there should be between two people.

Sometimes it is difficult for children to generate praise statements. Have children write down one or two praise statements next to the visual of the girl with the question mark.

Rules concretely specify prosocial behavior (e.g., listening to the person who is talking, body in space, appropriate gestures, etc.). Feel free to come back to this page in the workbook as needed, depending on what each learner needs.

In a one-on-one setting, this activity can be individualized to meet that child's needs.

Modifications

- Visual demonstration can be individualized to best suit the needs of the group (e.g., role-play, photographs, drawings, video modeling, songs, dance).

Box 4.2   Modifications for Social Skills Activities

Suggested modifications have been provided for each social skills activity. These modifications are changes that can be made to individualize the activities to different learners, to incorporate when the suggested materials are not available, and to provide accommodations.

Getting to Know New Friends: The ME Crest

The ME Crest (Session 1, Children's Workbook) involves children drawing things about themselves on a crest template and is meant to aid the group members in getting to know one another and encourage child participation (where the children can talk about themselves, their interests and strengths). The ME Crest is a **beginner** skill that helps children build communication skills, such as attending to others and following simple instructions, group skills, such as waiting a turn and remaining seated in a group, play skills, such as engaging in parallel play, and self-regulation, such as tolerating new rules and expectations.

Instructions: Ask children to complete the fill-in-the-blank questions in the workbook. Therapists can then show children their completed ME Crest and ask them to complete their own ME Crest and write down or draw things about themselves (see Me Crest in Session 1, Children's Workbook). Caregiver assistance may be needed.

Each child will then be encouraged to share their information. Reiterate that children can share as much or as little information as they would like. Give praise to children for sharing, and model appropriate back-and-forth conversation (by taking an interest and building on what they share). Deliver tokens as you feel appropriate.

In a one-on-one setting, the child may informally share their ME Crest with the therapist and/or caregivers.

Modifications

- Caregiver may discuss the fill-in-the-blank questions with their child and fill them out on their child's behalf.
- Children may also draw their answers.

Cheeky Chance

Cheeky Chance (Session 2, Children's Workbook) involves children taking turns rolling a die and choosing an activity to complete based on the number rolled (e.g., if a five is rolled and the child chooses jumping jacks, everyone will do five jumping jacks). Cheeky Chance is a **beginner** skill that helps children build communication skills, such as attending to others, and giving and following simple instructions, group skills, such as waiting a turn and remaining seated or standing in a group, play skills, such as engaging in cooperative play, and self-regulation, such as tolerating sharing and waiting.

Instructions: Explain that everyone is going to have a chance to roll the die and that the person who rolls gets to decide which activity everyone is going to play. The number on the die is the number of times the activity is played. For example, if a child rolls a six and they want to do jumping jacks, everyone will do six jumping jacks. If needed, demonstrate rolling the die and playing a game before the children take a turn. Both physical and non-physical activities should be encouraged. When the person has finished their turn, encourage everyone to give a high-five to the people next to them. Continue until everyone has had a turn.

In a one-on-one setting, the therapist and/or caregivers can participate in the activity by taking turns rolling the die and performing the actions alongside the child.

Modifications

- If dice aren't available, numbers can be drawn from a hat, or a physical or virtual number wheel can be used.

Collect, Pass, Run, and Sort – The Running Relay

The Collect, Pass, Run, and Sort – Running Relay (Session 3 and 7, Children's Workbook) involves children working together to complete a relay and scavenger hunt. This activity is an **intermediate** skill that helps children build communication skills, such as giving and following simple instructions, group skills, such as waiting a turn and following group instructions, play skills, such as engaging in sustained cooperative play, and self-regulation, such as tolerating sharing and waiting for longer periods of time.

Instructions: Place grocery item pictures around the room and mark the floor with prompts for where each child should stand according to their role (e.g., Passer, Runner, Sorter). Each picture corresponds with a corresponding picture in each child's grocery basket. In group therapy, inform the children to get into groups of three and assign each child with one of the three roles. Inform the children that the goal is to collect all the grocery items as a team using their designated roles. If needed, you can model the scavenger hunt. Say "On your mark, get set, GO!" to start the race. Prompt the children to encourage one another. Once all items have been retrieved and sorted, have the children switch roles and repeat the activity. If time permits, do this until each child has had a turn playing each of the three roles.

In a one-on-one setting, the therapist and caregiver may participate in the relay race with the child, or the child can perform the relay more than once and try to do it in the fastest time.

Modifications

- If a relay race isn't possible, a scavenger hunt or Eye-Spy game can be played instead.

Alphabet Game

The Alphabet Game (Session 4, Children's Workbook) requires children to move their bodies to mimic different letters of the alphabet. This activity is an **intermediate** skill that helps children build communication skills, such as giving and following more complex instructions, group skills, such as engaging in imitation within a group setting, play skills, such as engaging in sustained imaginative play, and self-regulation, such as tolerating periods waiting.

Instructions: Have the children stand in a circle. Inform the children that they will be making shapes using their bodies. Model the activity first by choosing a letter and using your body to make that shape. Encourage the children to copy you. Next, go around the circle so that each child has a turn to choose a letter and demonstrate the shape. Children can use the first letter of their name or choose their favorite letter. Encourage the children to copy each child as they demonstrate the shape. Continue until each child has had a turn.

In a one-on-one setting, the therapist and/or caregivers can participate in the activity by making the letters of the alphabet alongside the child.

Modifications

- Instead of letters, the children can act out animals, characters, vehicles, etc.
- Children can also take turns moving their bodies to different sounds (e.g., making a star shape with their body when they hear cymbals).

Drawing and Sharing Seasonal Pictures

Drawing and Sharing Seasonal Pictures (Session 4, Children's Workbook) involves children using various art mediums (e.g., crayons, markers, felt, construction paper) to create a seasonal picture. This activity is an **intermediate** skill that helps children build communication skills, such as describing picture scenes to peers, group skills, such as waiting a turn and engaging in a sustained group activity, play skills, such as engaging in sustained parallel play while creating their picture, and self-regulation, such as tolerating periods of uninterrupted play, as well as sharing and waiting for longer periods of time.

Instructions: Ask the children to think of what they like about this time of year (e.g., smelling flowers, going to the beach, jumping in leaf piles, building snowmen, depending on the season!). If group therapy, divide the children into small groups and provide each group with a set of art supplies to share (e.g., markers, stickers, stencils). Ask the children to use their imaginations to create a seasonal picture. Once everyone is finished, encourage each child to share their picture with their group. If a child is hesitant, they may show their picture to a therapist or another child. After each child has shown their picture, encourage the group to compliment them and share what they liked about their picture.

In a one-on-one setting, the child may informally share and discuss their picture with the therapist and/or caregivers.

Modifications

- Different topics can be incorporated instead of reasons, such as drawing their favorite characters, foods, activities, etc.
- Children can also create 3D models or structures using building materials (e.g., Play-Doh, popsicle sticks).

Freestyle Building

Freestyle Building (Session 5, Children's Workbook) requires children to work together to recreate an image using building blocks (e.g., LEGO®). This activity is an **intermediate** skill that helps children build communication skills, such as giving and following more complex instructions from peers, group skills, such as engaging in a sustained activity in a group, play skills, such as engaging in sustained cooperative play and helping others, and self-regulation, such as tolerating adapting to change and feedback from peers.

Instructions: Have the children get into pairs (Note: it may be helpful to have children with similar skill levels paired with one another). Give each pair a bag of construction materials and a picture. Next, tell the group they will be working together to recreate the picture using the construction materials they've been given. For children that build quickly, provide them with more complex pictures or multiple pictures to recreate. Once everyone is finished, encourage each pair to share their structures with the group. After each pair has shared their structure, encourage the group to congratulate them and share what they liked about their structure.

In a one-on-one setting, the child can complete the activity on their own, then share what they created.

Modifications

- Other materials can be used in place of construction materials, such as K'NEX®, Play-Doh®, or even marshmallows and toothpicks.

Building Our Greeting Bank

Building Our Greeting Bank (Session 6, Children's Workbook) involves children working together to think of a variety of ways to greet others.

This activity is an **intermediate** skill that helps children build communication skills, such as giving and following more complex instructions from peers, group skills, such as engaging in joint problem solving with peers, play skills, such as using imagination to think of scenarios, and self-regulation, such as tolerating adapting to change and feedback from peers.

Instructions: Bring the children over to the two masking tape ladders on the floor (there should be one ladder for every two children). Inform children to find a friend/partner to work with. For children who are reluctant, encourage/facilitate the initiation to choose a partner. Describe that the objective of the game is to stand on opposite sides of the greeting ladder and reach the center to collect play "money" for their greeting bank. Describe how this "money" can "buy" help when you and your partner are unsure of a way to show that you are proud of each other. Provide each pair with starter "money" (relative to the cost of help and how many ladder spaces there are). Provide examples of how the children can earn more "money". The children can only move forward one spot once each partner has practiced showing their friend one way they are proud of them. For example, each child can hop one step of the ladder when they have given their friend a thumbs-up, or each child can hop one step of the ladder when they have yelled "Great work!" Have a therapist and another adult model the same examples that were just described. On the third rung have the pair "buy" help from another adult. Tell the children to start climbing and building their greeting bank. Any remaining "money" can be exchanged for a token which they can put on their token board. Encourage the children to use the things learned today next time they are proud of their friend.

In a one-on-one setting, the therapist and/or caregivers can participate in creating the greetings with the child.

Modifications

• Both verbal and nonverbal greetings can be included.

Building Buddies

Building Buddies (Session 6, Children's Workbook) requires children to work together to construct a building. This activity is an **intermediate** skill that helps children build communication skills, such as giving and following more complex instructions from peers, group skills, such as engaging in a sustained activity within a group, play skills, such as engaging in sustained cooperative play and helping others, and self-regulation, such as tolerating adapting to change and feedback from peers.

Instructions: Ask the children to reflect on the Freestyle Building activity. Ask them what they built in that activity – this can help them think of similar things to build during this activity. Have the children get into groups of three (Note: it may be helpful to have children with similar skill levels grouped together). Let the group know that each child will have a special role in their small groups – Engineer, Supplier, and Builder. Model each of these three roles (e.g., sharing ideas as the Engineer, distributing the blocks as the Supplier, and putting pieces together as the Builder). Give each group a bag of building blocks (e.g., LEGO®) and name tags to remind each child of their role. Tell the children they can start creating a building of their choice. When everyone is finished, encourage each triad to share their buildings with the group. After each triad has shared their building, encourage the group to congratulate them and share what they liked about their building.

In a one-on-one setting, the child can be given the choice of completing the activity on their own, then sharing what they created, or working with the therapist and/or caregiver.

Modifications

• Other materials can be used in place of construction materials, such as K'NEX®, Play-Doh®, or even marshmallows and toothpicks.

Build and Borrow

Build and Borrow (Session 7, Children's Workbook) requires children to work together to construct a building and communicate with members of other groups. This activity is an **advanced** skill that helps children build communication skills, such as engaging in sustained conversation with peers, group skills, such as engaging in group problem solving, play skills, such as engaging in sustained cooperative play with peers and the larger group, and self-regulation, such as tolerating giving preferred items to others and expressing enthusiasm for others' success.

Instructions: Have the children get into pairs (Note: it may be helpful to have children with similar skill levels paired with one another). Give each pair a bag of building blocks (e.g., LEGO®) and a picture. Each bag of blocks only contains one style of block (e.g., Pair 1 has the blue blocks, Pair 2 has the red blocks, etc.). Tell the children they will be working in pairs to recreate the picture using the blocks they've been given. Ask the children what they notice about their bags of blocks and what they need to do to recreate their pictures (sharing their blocks with other groups). For children who build quickly, provide them with more complex pictures or multiple pictures to recreate. Once everyone is finished, encourage each pair to share their structures with the group. After each pair has shared their structure, encourage the group to congratulate them and share what they liked about their structure.

In a one-on-one setting, the child can be given the choice of completing the activity on their own, then sharing what they created, or completing the activity cooperatively with the therapist and/or their caregivers.

Modifications

• Other materials can be used in place of construction materials, such as K'NEX®, Play-Doh®, or even marshmallows and toothpicks.

Share-A-Way

Share-A-Way (Session 8, Children's Workbook) involves children sharing information and listening while others share information. This activity is an **advanced** skill that helps children build communication skills, such as engaging in sustained conversation with peers, group skills, such as listening to information being shared to the larger group, play skills, such as engaging in sustained cooperative play with peers and the larger group, and self-regulation, such as tolerating giving preferred items to others and expresses enthusiasm for others' success.

Instructions: Break children into groups of two. Instruct the children to take out their item for sharing. Model appropriate behavior to the children by sharing your item first. Prompt the children to begin sharing their item with their partner. Once children have shared with their partner, have the children share with the larger group.

In a one-on-one setting, the child may informally share and discuss their item with the therapist and/or caregivers.

Modifications

• Children can share information about their favorite toys, TV shows, characters, foods, etc.

Picture Prep

Picture Prep (Session 8, Children's Workbook) requires children to practice taking turns and attending to others. This activity is an **advanced** skill that helps children build communication skills, such as engaging in sustained conversation with peers, group skills, such as listening to information being shared to the larger group, play skills, such as engaging in sustained cooperative play with peers and the larger group, and self-regulation, such as tolerating giving preferred items to others and expresses enthusiasm for others' success.

Instructions: Ask the children what they will need to take pictures with their friends. Facilitate having the children ask their peers to take a picture together. Prompt children who are waiting for a turn to write down ideas of what they'd like to do in their pictures.

In a one-on-one setting, the child can create their picture independently, with a preferred activity (e.g., their construction project).

Modifications

- If children can't have their photo taken, they can create a drawing of themselves or print a photo of their favorite character.

Picture Perfect

Picture Perfect (Session 9, Children's Workbook) requires children to reflect on what they have learned and create a memorable item that they can take with them after the program ends. This activity is an **advanced** skill that helps children build communication skills, such as engaging in sustained conversation with peers, group skills, such as listening to information being shared to the larger group, play skills, such as engaging in sustained cooperative play with peers and the larger group, and self-regulation, such as tolerating giving preferred items to others and expresses enthusiasm for others' success.

Instructions: Lay the photos from the previous week out on a table. Ask the children to come up and find their photos. Then, have the children gather up any art supplies that they might need and facilitate children working on making a card for a friend/instructor, or a picture to remember the group.

In a one-on-one setting, the child may informally share and discuss their picture with the therapist and/or caregivers.

Modifications

- Keywords, drawings, or pictures can be used to help children remember the activities they completed over the past nine weeks. If children don't have a photo the previous week, they can draw their experiences instead.

References

American Psychiatric Association. (2022). *Diagnostic and statistical manual of mental disorders* (5th ed., text rev.). https://doi.org/10.1176/appi.books.9780890425787

Barrett, P. M. (1998). Evaluation of cognitive-behavior group treatments for childhood anxiety disorders. *Journal of Clinical Child Psychology, 27*(4), 459–468. https://doi.org/10.1207/s15374424jccp2704_10

Bauminger, N. (2002). The facilitation of social-emotional understanding and social interaction in high-functioning children with autism: Intervention outcomes. *Journal of Autism and Developmental Disorders, 32*(4), 283–298. https://doi.org/10.1023/a:1016378718278

Bauminger, N. (2007). Brief report: Individual social-multi-modal intervention for HFASD. *Journal of Autism and Developmental Disorders, 37*(8), 1593–1604. https://doi.org/10.1007/s10803-006-0245-4

Beaumont, R., & Sofronoff, K. (2008). A multi-component social skills intervention for children with Asperger syndrome: The junior detective training program. *Journal of Child Psychology and Psychiatry, and Allied Disciplines, 49*(7), 743–753. https://doi.org/10.1111/j.1469-7610.2008.01920.x

Boyd, B. A., McDonough, S. G., & Bodfish, J. W. (2012). Evidence-based behavioral interventions for repetitive behaviors in autism. *Journal of Autism and Developmental Disorders, 42*(6), 1236–1248. https://doi.org/10.1007/s10803-011-1284-z

Boyd, B. A., Woodard, C. R., & Bodfish, J. W. (2013). Feasibility of exposure response prevention to treat repetitive behaviors of children with autism and an intellectual disability: A brief report. *Autism: The International Journal of Research and Practice, 17*(2), 196–204. https://doi.org/10.1177/1362361311414066

Cobham, V. E., Spence, S. H., & Dadds, M. R. (1998). The role of parental anxiety in the treatment of childhood anxiety. *Journal of Consulting and Clinical Psychology, 66*(6), 893–905. https://doi.org/10.1037/0022-006X.66.6.893

Cummins, C., Pellicano, E., & Crane, L. (2020). Autistic adults' views of their communication skills and needs. *International Journal of Language & Communication Disorders, 55*(5), 678–689. https://doi.org/10.1111/1460-6984.12552

Frankel, F., Myatt, R., Sugar, C., Whitham, C., Gorospe, C. M., & Laugeson, E. (2010). A randomized controlled study of parent-assisted children's friendship training with children having autism spectrum disorders. *Journal of Autism and Developmental Disorders, 40*(7), 827–842. https://doi.org/10.1007/s10803-009-0932-z

Guertin, E. L., Vause, T., Jaksic, H., Frijters, J. C., & Feldman, M. (2019). Treating obsessive compulsive behavior and enhancing peer engagement in a preschooler with intellectual disability. *Behavioral Interventions, 34*(1), 19–29. https://doi.org/10.1002/bin.1646

Harrop, C., McBee, M., & Boyd, B. A. (2016). How are child restricted and repetitive behaviors associated with caregiver stress over time? A parallel process multilevel growth model. *Journal of Autism and Developmental Disorders, 46*(5), 1773–1783. https://doi.org/10.1007/s10803-016-2707-7

Howard, P. L., & Sedgewick, F. (2021). 'Anything but the phone!': Communication mode preferences in the autism community. *Autism, 25*(8), 2265–2278. https://doi.org/10.1177/13623613211014995

Krempa, J., & McKinnon, K. (2002). *Social skills solutions: A hands-on manual for teaching social skills to children with autism.* DRL Books, Inc.

Lawrence, H. (2023, June 5). *Neurodiversity affirming approaches to teaching social skills.* Twinkl. https://www.twinkl.ca/blog/neurodiversity-affirming-approaches-to-teaching-social-skills

Manassis, K., Lee, T. C., Bennett, K., Zhao, X. Y., Mendlowitz, S., Duda, S., Saini, M., Wilansky, P., Baer, S., Barrett, P., Bodden, D., Cobham, V. E., Dadds, M. R., Flannery-Schroeder, E., Ginsburg, G., Heyne, D., Hudson, J. L., Kendall, P. C., Liber, J., Masia-Warner, C., . . . Wood, J. J. (2014). Types of parental involvement in CBT with anxious youth: A preliminary meta-analysis. *Journal of Consulting and Clinical Psychology, 82*(6), 1163–1172. https://doi.org/10.1037/a0036969

Martin, G., & Pear, J. J. (2024). *Behavior modification: What is it and how to do it* (12th ed.). Routledge.

Mathur, S. K., Renz, E., & Tarbox, J. (2024). Affirming neurodiversity within applied behavior analysis. *Behavior Analysis in Practice, 17*, 471–485. https://doi.org/10.1007/s40617-024-00907-3

Noell, G. H., Call, N. A., & Ardoin. S. P. (2014). Building complex repertoires from discrete behaviors by establishing stimulus control, behavioral chains, and strategic behavior. In W. W. Fisher, C. C. Piazza, & H. S. Roane (Eds.), *Handbook of applied behavior analysis* (pp. 250–269). Guildford Press.

Partington, J. W. (2006). *The assessment of basic language and learning skills-revised.* Pleasant Hill.

Patel, S. P., Landau, E., Martin, G. E., Rayburn, C., Elahi, S., Fragnito, G., & Losh, M. (2023). A profile of prosodic speech differences in individuals with autism spectrum disorder and first-degree relatives. *Journal of Communication Disorders, 102*, 106313. https://doi.org/10.1016/j.jcomdis.2023.106313

Sundberg, M. L. (2008). *Verbal behavior milestones assessment and placement program.* AVB Press.

Vause, T., Neil, N., & Feldman, M. (2020). Functional behavior-based cognitive-behavioral therapy for obsessive-compulsive behavior in children with ASD. In F. R. Volkmar (Ed.), *Encyclopedia of autism spectrum disorders.* Springer. https://doi.org/10.1007/978-1-4614-6435-8_102481-1

Wise, S. J. (2023, May 14). *Neurodiversity affirming practice: Core principles.* Medium. https://medium.com/@livedexperienceeducator/neurodiversity-affirming-practice-core-principles-f2c6d70661af

Wood, J. J., Fujii, C., & Renno, P. (2010). Cognitive behavioral therapy in high-functioning autism: Review and recommendations for treatment development. In B. Reichow, P. Doehring, D. Cicchetti, & F. Volkmar (Eds.), *Evidence-based practices and treatments for children with autism* (pp. 197–230). Springer.

Zablotsky, B., Bradshaw, C. P., Anderson, C. M., & Law, P. (2013). Risk factors for bullying among children with autism spectrum disorders. *Autism, 18*(4), 419–427. https://doi.org/10.1177/1362361313477920

Chapter 5

Considerations for Running Sessions

Individual and Group Therapy

Chapter 1 details the evidence supporting functional behavior-based cognitive behavioral therapy (Fb-CBT) as group therapy including our randomized controlled trial (RCT) study. In our RCT, we ran Fb-CBT with two therapists and multiple children. Throughout the sessions, we discuss how each session can be run as both individual and group therapy. To this end, comments are made throughout each component in Sessions 1 through 9 regarding group and individual formats.

Timing

Each session in the RCT was two hours, run in a group format, and we have provided a recommended time frame for each component based on this session length and format. For **individual therapy**, we assume therapists will adjust the various components to fit the client. Please be mindful that our timings are only approximations. Based on therapist and client preference, you may choose to do the activities in a different order or spend less or more time on them. Note that for Sessions 2 through 9, the 25-minute caregiver module may run at the same time as two child activities. Refer to the caregiver module column in Table 5.1.

Assessing and Administering Different Components of Fb-CBT Based on Your Background

Therapists who use Fb-CBT come from a variety of backgrounds. If you are a behavior analyst, you may refer to Chapter 3 on functional behavior assessments (FBAs) but likely already have a system in place. If you have a limited behavioral background, you may need to read Chapter 3 in more detail and follow the assessments provided. We've designed the FBA component such that you conduct your functional assessment and then give the caregiver a user-friendly intervention that will become increasingly familiar to them as

DOI: 10.4324/9781003410126-5

they work through obsessive-compulsive behaviors (OCBs) and caregiver modules. Likewise, if your strengths are in cognitive behavioral therapy (CBT), you likely will follow the CBT pieces, doing what works from your own experience. Last, we have designed a progressive social skills sequence; as a therapist, you may choose what works for the children and youth that you serve. You may follow the examples verbatim or use them as a guide.

Clinical Assessment and Collecting Caregiver Data

Prior to beginning Session 1, conduct a clinical assessment of the child or youth's OCBs. Clinical assessments and data collection can be conducted in a variety of ways (see Chapter 2 for a detailed example from our RCT). Therapists should use their professional judgment when choosing which ones to use. In Chapter 2, we have provided (a) a data-sheet to record the child's obsessions and compulsions, (b) a datasheet to assess the level of interference to determine targeted OCBs and gather information about them, and (c) a user-friendly (Likert scale) caregiver rating form to collect weekly data on OCBs. Additional assessments not included in Chapter 2 may be used based on the therapist's judgment.

Feasibility of Data Collection and Criteria in Each Session for Addressing New OCBs

It is ideal to obtain some data from caregivers on their child's OCBs before Session 1. If this is not feasible, begin collecting caregiver data when Session 1 begins. In the RCT and clinical practice, we often had caregivers collect data three days per week (e.g., every Monday, Wednesday, and Friday); some caregivers collected data daily. This is a conversation to have with each caregiver to assess what is feasible in addition to support-ing and encouraging their child throughout treatment. Keep in mind that you can assess progress with other forms of data (e.g., the stimulus map and Exposure/Response Prevention [E/RP] sheets beginning in Session 3).

This data will help you make informed decisions about each child's progress and when to introduce a new OCB into treatment. Regarding treating new OCBs, we have developed criteria based on minimal and good progress. You can use this as a guide and tailor the requirements of each learner as appropriate.

Overview of Sessions

Table 5.1 presents an overview of all sessions. It includes (a) session topics, (b) caregiver modules, (c) guidelines for adding new OCBs, (d) social skills activities, and (d) tasks therapists need to complete to

Table 5.1 Overview of Sessions and Caregiver Modules

Session	Topic	Caregiver Module	Guidelines for Adding New OCBs	Social Skills Activities	Therapist Preparation for Upcoming Session
1	Session Expectations, Rapport Building, and Introduction to Psychoeducation	Overview of Caregiver Modules To take place at the end of session	No OCBs added	1. Session Rules 2. Getting to Know New Friends: The ME Crest	• Schedule FBA appointments with caregivers (if possible)
2	Learning About Obsessions, Being the Boss, and Mapping of OCBs	The OCB Cycle * Schedule FBA appointment for the coming week To take place during Break and Snack, and Designing a Fear Thermometer	No OCBs added	1. Cheeky Chance	• Complete pre-planning CBT Skills Template • Schedule FBA appointments • Complete FBA and Competing Behavior Model • Complete FBAI for the first OCB
3	CBT Skills Training and Beginning E/RP for First OCB	Introduction to Functional Behavior Assessment and FBAI To take place during Break and Snack, and Collect, Pass, Run, and Sort – The Running Relay	OCB #1 added	1. Collect, Pass, Run, and Sort – The Running Relay	• Review three sample E/RP Worksheets • Complete pre-planning CBT Skills Template • Complete FBA with caregiver to inform FBAI for the next OCB
4	Progress Review of First OCB and Tackling New OCBs	Functional Behavior Assessment and FBAI: Special Topic on Setting Events To take place during Break and Snack, and Drawing and Sharing a Seasonal Picture	Developing Fluency: Review OCB #1 and Program for OCB #2 * Encourage Generalization	1. Alphabet Game 2. Drawing and Sharing a Seasonal Picture	• Complete pre-planning CBT Skills Template • Prepare FBAI for the next OCB

(Continued)

Table 5.1 (Continued)

Session	Topic	Caregiver Module	Guidelines for Adding New OCBs	Social Skills Activities	Therapist Preparation for Upcoming Session
5	Continued OCB Mapping and Gradually Moving Up the Hierarchy	Functional Behavior Assessment and FBAI: Special Topic on Addressing Dual Functions. To take place during Break and Snack, and Freestyle Building	Developing Fluency: Review OCB #2 and Program for OCB #3 * Encourage Generalization	1. Freestyle Building	• Complete CBT Skills Template • Prepare FBAI for the next OCB
6	Relapse Prevention and Introducing More Flexibility with OCBs	Exposure and Response Prevention: Choosing E/RP Steps. To take place during Break and Snack, and Building Buddies	Developing Fluency: Review OCB #3 and Program for OCB #4 and possibly 5 * Encourage Generalization	1. Building Our Greeting Bank 2. Building Buddies	• Complete CBT Skills Template • Prepare FBAIs for next OCBs
7	Relapse Prevention, Generalization, and Introducing More Flexibility with OCBs	Introduction to Reinforcement. To take place during Break and Snack, and Build and Borrow	Review Previous OCBs, add OCBs as appropriate from the same and different response classes	1. Collect, Pass, Run, and Sort – The Running Relay 2. Build and Borrow	• Complete CBT Skills Template • Prepare FBAIs for next OCBs
8	Relapse Prevention, Generalization, and Tackling Final OCBs	Reinforcement Thinning. To take place during Break and Snack, and Picture Prep	Review Previous OCBs, Add OCBs as appropriate from the same and different response classes	1. Share-A-Way 2. Picture Prep	• Complete CBT Skills Template • Prepare FBAIs for next OCBs
9	Revisiting Quality of Life, Wrap-Up, and Graduation	Wrap-Up, Review, and Reflection. To take place during Break and Snack, and Picture Perfect	Review Previous OCBs, and Program for OCBs if Desired **Booster Sessions	1. Picture Perfect	If needed: • Schedule follow-up FBA • Prepare materials for Booster Sessions

* Check for re-emergence of tackled OCBs and program as appropriate.
** Remember to schedule weekly FBA appointments (to complete the functional behavior assessment and intervention [FBAI]) in Caregiver Modules.

prepare for upcoming sessions. Session 1 begins with an introduction to the expectations of the group, the workbook, and establishing rapport, followed by psychoeducation on OCBs. Psychoeducation continues in Session 2, and a fear thermometer and stimulus mapping of OCBs are introduced. In Session 3, children are introduced to cognitive and behavioral skills training and select their first OCB to begin E/RP. Sessions 4 to 6 include reviewing progress for OCBs that have begun E/RP and introducing additional OCBs if appropriate. Sessions 7, 8, and 9 focus on programming for flexibility and relapse prevention. Graduation takes place at the end of Session 9.

Finally, bold text in the sessions refers to materials provided in the manual or activities in the Children's Workbook. Italics refer to language the therapist can say to the children. These words are not meant to be memorized or used verbatim but provided as guidance.

Chapter 6

Session 1

Expectations, Rapport Building, and Introduction to Psychoeducation

---

Materials

- Children's Workbook
- Name tags (optional)
- Flipchart/Whiteboard
- Token board (Session 1, Appendix A)
- Tokens and a bag or bin of preferred items
- Completed Reinforcer Checklist (Chapter 1, Appendix B)
- Activities/food for break and snack
- ABC Narrative Form (Chapter 3, Appendix B)
- Therapist completed ME Crest (from Children's Workbook)
- Obsession and Compulsion Recording Template (Chapter 2, Appendix B)
- Operational Definitions and Interference Handout (Chapter 2, Appendix C)

Session Outline

- General Welcome and Introductions (10 Min.)
- Introduce the Visual Schedule (5 Min.)
- Introduce the Children's Workbook (5 Min.)
- Social Skills Activity: Session Rules (10 Min.)
- Rewarding Positive Behavior: Token Exchange (10 Min.)
- Break and Snack (10 Min.)
- Social Skills Activity: Getting to Know New Friends: The ME Crest (15 Min.)
- Our Strengths and Challenges (10 Min.)
- What Is Obsessive-Compulsive Behavior? (25 Min.)
- Assigning Homework (5 Min.)
- Token Exchange and Goodbyes (5 Min.)
- Caregiver Module 1: Overview of Caregiver Modules (10 Min.) – To take place at the end of session

DOI: 10.4324/9781003410126-6

Pre-Session Checklist

Arranging the Environment

- Arrange the seating in the room so it is comfortable and accessible. For group therapy, furniture can be arranged to resemble a circle, square, or other suitable configuration. Ensure there is ample space to divide into caregiver/child dyads and for you (the therapist) to engage in conversation with each dyad.
- Before each session, outline activities on a whiteboard or flipchart using the workbook session schedule. This will allow the child to see the sequence of activities planned for the session. You can even check off each activity when it is complete.
- Many autistic children have difficulty communicating vocally and transitioning from one activity to another. A visual schedule provides structure and predictability for the therapy sessions and presents it in a manner that is accessible for learners with difficulty understanding spoken words. Pictures or other visuals may be used instead of text when applicable or desired. For more information on these adaptations, see Chapter 1 (Appendix A: Adaptations to Support Autistic Children).

Caregiver Data Sheets

- If caregivers were asked to collect data before Session 1, collect these caregiver data sheets at the beginning of this session or during the scheduled break. Blank **Caregiver Weekly Data Forms** and a completed sample are in Chapter 2 (Appendix E: Blank Caregiver Weekly Data Form).
- Briefly review each completed **Caregiver Weekly Data Form** to get an idea of behaviors the child has some control over, and others that are more difficult. Obtain the child and caregiver's input as often as needed. Use these sheets as a guide for children's exercises when discussing obsessive-compulsive behaviors (OCBs) and whether the child can resist OCB sometimes or not at all. The purpose of doing this is to collect information to determine the first OCB to address.

Session Implementation

General Welcome and Introductions

In group therapy, participating members (children, caregivers, therapists) may choose to wear a nametag. Therapists will begin by welcoming all group members. As a therapist, introduce yourself first and describe what your role will be. Then, encourage children and caregivers to introduce themselves. Ask them to say their names and any other information they would like to share (e.g., their pronouns) and anything about themselves (e.g., their likes or dislikes).

Be mindful that children may be nervous, especially in the first session. Caregivers may be nervous too! Emphasize that each person may share as little or as much as they would like, using their modality of choice (see Chapter 1 for more information on concrete versus abstract learners, child voice, and anxiety).

Autistic children may have trouble engaging and communicating in social situations. For example, a child may have difficulty listening to the speaker and taking turns with others. A bean bag (or other visual) can be used as a tangible cue (also known as a prompt) to signal when it is the child's turn to listen and when it is their turn to speak. Direct eye contact with the speaker is not necessary. Do your best to encourage learners to orient towards the speaker in a manner that is comfortable for them. Offering sensory toys or games or allowing the child to bring one from home may reduce their anxiety or help them focus.

For individual therapy, having a visual or manipulative as a cue for who is talking may also be useful. It can be a fun activity and a way to keep children engaged, too. A bin of sensory toys may be beneficial and can be helpful calming tools for children.

Introduce the Visual Schedule

Refer to the list of activities outlined on the whiteboard/flipchart that align with the **Children's Workbook**. Draw a box next to each activity that can be checked off when each one is complete. Introduce the visual schedule using clear and simple language. Children often like to be the ones to check off the items. If this is the case, encourage their participation to foster engagement and awareness of the schedule.

Clear and simple language when talking to autistic learners often aids in comprehension. Use short and simple sentences. Of course, this may not be the case for all learners. See Chapter 1 (concrete versus abstract learners; Table 1 on Adaptations to Support Autistic Children) for more details.

Introduce the Children's Workbook

Give each child their copy of the **Children's Workbook**. Explain that they will be using the workbook throughout the nine treatment sessions.

Some sections will be completed in session, and others will be completed at home. It is important to communicate to learners that this is their workbook; they can mark it up in any way they would like (e.g., using pencils, pens, markers, stickers). Also, when the sessions are completed, the workbook can be taken home and referred to as needed.

Social Skills Activity: Session Rules

Session rules are used to establish session expectations. This is a beginner social skill activity (see Chapter 4 for further details on the social skills curriculum).

Instructions: Ask each child to turn to the page in their workbook that has a set of "session rules" to follow. These should be reviewed for both group and individual therapy. Explain why we need rules and read each rule (or have children read the rules aloud). Use role-playing with the visuals in the workbook to provide a visual demonstration of each rule. If children are willing, have them read the rules aloud, and participate in role-playing. For example, you may read the rule "keep your hands and feet to yourselves and respect the personal space of others" and have the members do an exercise where they put their arms out and turn around in a circle. You can indicate that this is how much space there should be between two people.

Sometimes it is difficult for children to generate praise statements. Have children write down one or two praise statements next to the visual of the girl with the question mark.

Rules concretely specify prosocial behavior (e.g., listening to the person who is talking, body in space, appropriate gestures, etc.). Feel free to come back to this sheet in the workbook as needed.

In a one-on-one setting, this activity can be individualized to meet that child's needs. See Chapter 4 for additional modifications.

Rewarding Positive Behavior: Token Exchange

A token economy is a commonly used behavior analytic technique. A token economy can help increase prosocial behaviors and requires three basic elements: tokens or small, countable items, clearly defined behaviors, and a backup reinforcer. A backup reinforcer is an item or activity the tokens can be exchanged for. Additional information is presented in Chapter 1 (Positive Reinforcement).

Use a preference assessment, such as the sample reinforcer checklist provided (Chapter 1; Appendix B) or the Reinforcement Assessment for Individuals with Severe Developmental Disabilities (Chapter 2), to determine preferred items to use as backup reinforcers. These would preferably be completed before treatment begins.

Present each child with a token sheet. When explaining what it is for, direct children to the visual in the workbook labeled **Token Exchange**. Explain how tokens can be earned (e.g., following rules, participating in activities, or saying something nice to a person), and when/what they can be traded in for. Write down target prosocial behaviors (with the assistance of children/caregivers) on their token board. Explain that when you see them engaging in any of these behaviors, they will earn a token. Therapists should attempt to deliver one token to each child for prosocial behavior and by the end of the session, children should have earned all ten tokens.

Whenever possible, incorporate individual interests and preferences. For example, if a child expresses that they like spaceships, they could receive spaceship stickers, or the stickers could be placed inside a picture of a spaceship. There are ten spots on the token sheet (see Appendix A: Token Board).

A live demonstration can support the visual aid in the workbook. To do this, the therapist can request that someone (child or caregiver) demonstrate a prosocial behavior (e.g., saying a positive comment to another individual), and then the therapist delivers a token that the child places on their token board.

Have a **grab bag** available at the end of the session with several "mystery" prizes inside. From our experience, children liked it when the items were individually wrapped; it added an additional surprise! Explain that when the token sheet is complete, the children can exchange their tokens for an item from the grab bag. This exchange should be done at the end of each session. It can be helpful to have the grab bags visible but out of reach during sessions.

Some children may choose not to engage in the token exchange. Instead, they may engage in self-monitoring of predetermined behaviors that could be exchanged for an item, activity, or social opportunity of their choice.

Break and Snack

Before each session, ensure you ask about allergies and dietary restrictions. You may select snacks from the **Reinforcer Checklist** (see Chapter 1, Appendix B). Depending on your policies, snacks may be prepared ahead of time, or caregivers may be asked to bring in snacks.

You may use this time to observe OCBs or contrive situations to collect descriptive data (if possible) using the **ABC Narrative Form** (Chapter 3, Appendix B), or you may use one of your own.

Allow this break period to be child-directed (e.g., a child may want to draw or attempt to initiate a game with you). You can capitalize on this time to build rapport with the children or facilitate rapport building within the group. If helpful, use a timer and give children reminders of the time remaining.

Transitions from preferred activities can be difficult for many individuals with autism. Using a visual timer can assist children by showing them the passage of time and how much longer they have for an activity.

Social Skills Activity: Getting to Know New Friends: The ME Crest

This exercise is meant to aid the group members in getting to know one another and encourage child participation (where the children can talk about themselves, their interests, and strengths). This is a beginner social skill activity (see Chapter 4 for further details on the social skills curriculum).

Instructions: Ask children to complete fill-in-the-blank questions in the workbook activity: **The Me Crest: Getting to Know New Friends**. Therapists can then show children their completed ME Crest (completed prior to or during the session) and ask them to complete their own ME Crest and write down or draw things about themselves. Caregiver assistance may be needed.

Each child will then be encouraged to share their information. Reiterate that children can share as much or as little information as they would like. Give praise to children for sharing, and model appropriate back-and-forth conversation (by taking an interest and building on what they share). Deliver tokens as you feel appropriate.

In a one-on-one setting, the child may informally share their ME Crest with the therapist and/or caregivers. See Chapter 4 for additional modifications.

Our Strengths and Challenges

Referring to the workbook page titled **Our Strengths and Challenges**, focus on the key point that all of us are unique and have strengths as well as challenges. Give a simple definition of strengths. For example, *a strength is something that you do well and that you are proud of.* Refer children to examples in the workbook of different strengths. Then, have children write or draw one or more of their strengths with caregiver assistance, if needed. Encourage children to share this information if they feel comfortable.

Many of the activities throughout functional behavior-based cognitive behavioral therapy (Fb-CBT) provide various ways of communicating information (such as writing or drawing). Choices can help minimize challenging behavior due to tasks being difficult or requiring too much response effort.

Next, provide a simple definition of challenges. For example, *a challenge is something that we struggle with and often we need the help of others.* Go over the examples in the workbook. Ask the child to write or draw one challenge of their own.

Explain that by believing in ourselves and using our strengths, we can overcome our challenges.

Tell the group, *we are here today to discuss a common challenge we will work on. Lots of children have this challenge. It is called obsessive-compulsive behavior.*

What Is Obsessive-Compulsive Behavior?

Emphasize to the child that OCB is not his/her fault; it just happens. Relate OCB to the uncontrollable nature of pins and needles (see **What is Obsessive-Compulsive Behavior?** in the workbook to support explaining this concept).

Then, refer **to The OCB Story** in the workbook to explain that the brain sends out correct and incorrect messages. Read the different sections of the story and have the children follow along in the workbook. Support the explanation with visual cues (e.g., additional pictures on the whiteboard), if needed. You could also enlarge the workbook images and use them as visuals on the board or flip chart. Ask questions along the way to ensure children are comprehending the story.

Emphasize to children that they will learn new skills to help them recognize the incorrect messages that OCB sends. You want to convey that by believing in oneself, a child can fight OCB and those incorrect messages. Let the children know how strong they are by referring to the strengths they identified earlier (see Psychoeducation and Stimulus Mapping in Chapter 1).

As a brief exercise, have the children look at phrases written in **The OCB Story** in the workbook. Explain that these are some things you can say to OCB when it comes around. Then, have children write down alternative phrases that are meaningful to them. Praise children for taking the initiative to communicate the statements in their preferred modality and ask caregivers to do the same.

Many autistic children either do not have accompanying obsessions or have difficulty describing thoughts and feelings. We recommend encouraging learners to express associated thoughts, feelings, or worries, but not all individuals will do so. For more information, see Chapter 1, Complexity of Treating OCBs in Autism.

Turn to the workbook page on **Compulsions**. As an adaptation of Fb-CBT, we break OCB down into chunks. Explain that "B" stands for behavior. Then, explain that the "C" stands for compulsions. An explanation for compulsions might be: *Compulsions are actions that OCB makes us think we need to do. We often do them over and over again. We might do them because they help us stop worrying or feel safe. Sometimes we do them because they help us to feel good or just right. Regardless, they often take up lots of time or prevent us from doing things that we like to do with family and friends.*

Go over the examples of compulsions with the group. When discussing compulsions within the diagram, you may provide some examples of the children's compulsions from your pre-assessments and the **Obsession and Compulsion Recording Template** (Chapter 2, Appendix B) or they may volunteer things that they do. Caregivers can also actively participate in this process.

The next step is to have the children identify and describe their compulsions in their workbooks using the space provided in the **Compulsions** section. This may be a work in progress. Caregiver assistance or prompts may be needed, but over time, the children may need less support and get better at describing their compulsions. Have the **Obsession and Compulsion Recording Template** (Chapter 2, Appendix B) and the **Operational Definitions and Interference Handout** (Chapter 2, Appendix C) from the clinical assessment available. Attempt to have children think of compulsions on their own, but if they are having trouble generating examples, encourage them to use the sheets as a guide. As the therapist, provide the child with the level of assistance they need. In a group format, encourage children to share their compulsions with group members; if there are commonalities between group members, comment on this. Give children praise and tokens for sharing their thoughts and behaviors. Ultimately, you want the children to see that they are in a safe place to share their thoughts and feelings.

After listing compulsions, communicate to children that they are here to learn how to beat OCB and not have to worry or feel the urge to do their compulsions.

Assigning Homework

Briefly go over **How Can I Believe in Me Not OCB?** in the workbook that mentions the use of cognitive behavior therapy (CBT). It's now time to wrap up and assign homework. See the **Do-Think-Feel** exercise. Encourage children to write down at least two compulsions that happen before the next session. Ask caregivers to provide the assistance needed for children to begin to increase awareness of these compulsions (and accompanying thoughts, if present). Second, have children identify what parts of their body may feel different or uncomfortable when they feel the urge to do a compulsion. They can write down their feelings or color in parts of the body that felt uncomfortable or where there was a physiological sensation (e.g., heart beating faster). Last, ask each child to think of a nasty nickname for OCB and externalizing thoughts.

When finished, have children write down items that they need to bring to Session 2.

This homework activity encourages learners to identify the connection between behavior, thoughts, and emotions/sensations. As many children with autism have difficulty expressing internal states, we have found that children may return this worksheet partially completed. We continue to encourage identifying the relationship between behavior (Doing), thoughts (Thinking), and emotions (Feeling) as the sessions progress.

Token Exchange and Goodbyes

Before starting the token exchange, make sure you have the appropriate materials prepared (e.g., token sheet, stickers, grab bag of preferred items). Allow each child to exchange their tokens for a grab-bag item of their choosing. After each child has chosen an item, encourage them to say goodbye to one another (if run in a group format). This may need to be modeled and prompted for the first few sessions.

Note: At this point, the caregivers will complete Caregiver Module 1: Overview of Caregiver Modules (10 Min.).

Caregiver Module 1: Overview of Caregiver Modules

Distribute new **Caregiver Weekly Data Forms** (Chapter 2, Appendix E). Explain to caregivers that beginning in Session 2, a 25-minute caregiver module will be included within each two-hour session. Modules will cover topics like the OCB cycle, functional variables that may maintain OCBs beyond anxiety, and applied exercises to practice various

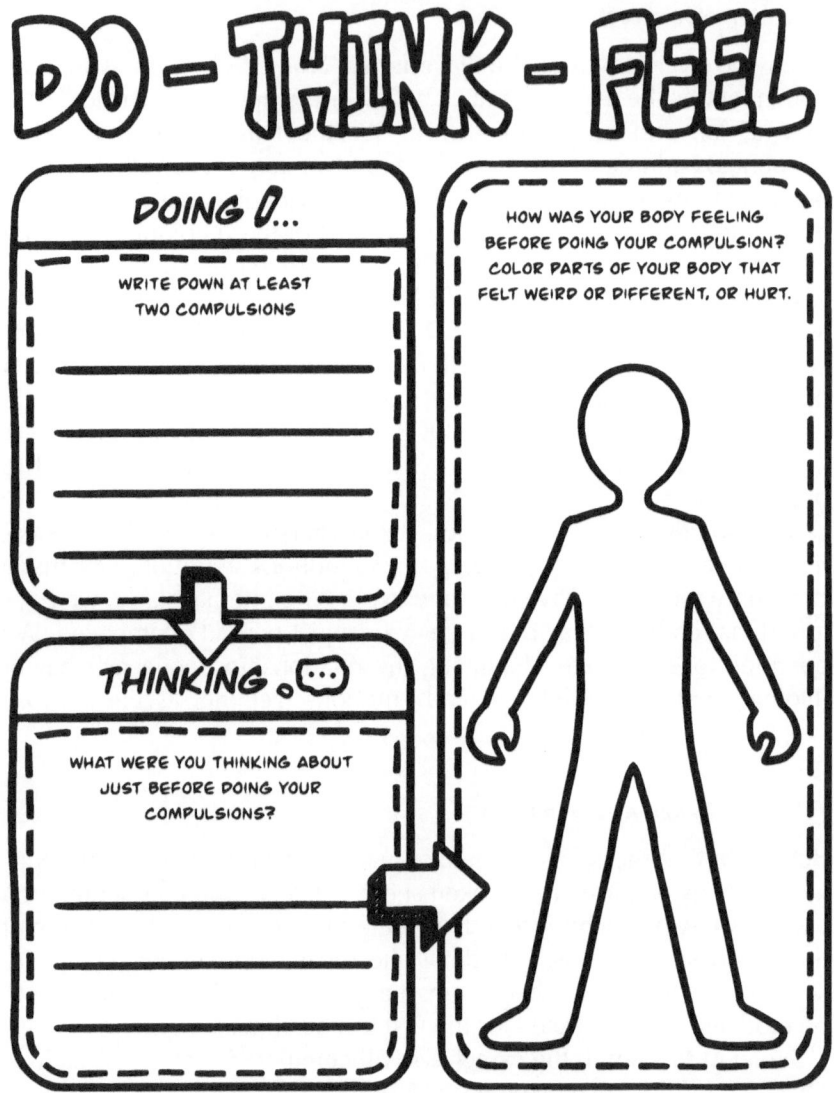

DO - THINK - FEEL

DOING

WRITE DOWN AT LEAST
TWO COMPULSIONS

THINKING

WHAT WERE YOU THINKING ABOUT
JUST BEFORE DOING YOUR
COMPULSIONS?

HOW WAS YOUR BODY FEELING
BEFORE DOING YOUR COMPULSION?
COLOR PARTS OF YOUR BODY THAT
FELT WEIRD OR DIFFERENT, OR HURT.

IT'S OK TO JUST WRITE DOWN YOUR COMPULSIONS. YOU MAY NOT
HAVE FEELINGS OR THOUGHTS THAT GO WITH THEM.

Figure 6.1 Do-Think-Feel exercise.

treatment strategies (e.g., addressing functional variables, choosing exposure steps, differentiating and fading reinforcers). Using behavioral skills training, the goal is to gradually transfer the strategies from therapist to caregiver, so they can act as a coach or supporter for their child and promote child independence as much as possible.

Explain that you will contact them to administer a brief functional assessment between Sessions 2 and 3. This will take approximately 30 minutes and can be done via telephone, videoconference, or in person. Explain that this will enable you to design a key piece of the intervention plan called the functional behavioral assessment and intervention (FBAI). If time permits, you may want to begin scheduling the appointments in this session or before Session 2.

Token Board

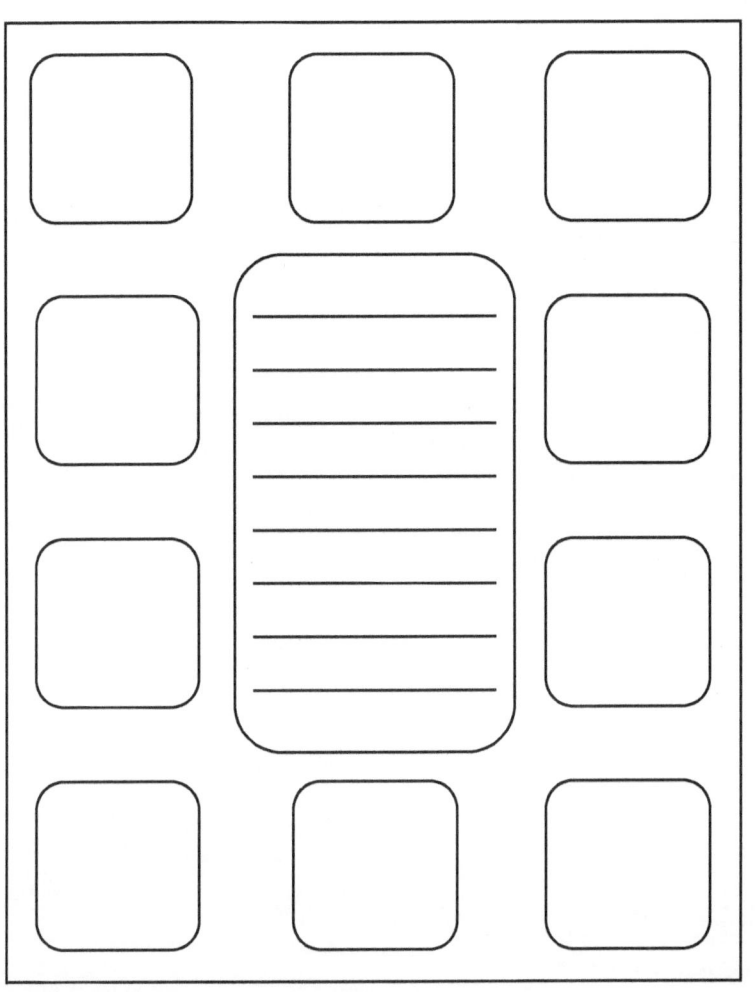

Chapter 7

Session 2

Learning About Obsessions, Being the Boss, and Mapping of OCBs

Materials

- Children's Workbook
- Flipchart/Whiteboard
- Caregiver Weekly Data Form (Chapter 2, Appendix E)
- Token Board (Session 1, Appendix A)
- Tokens and a bag or bin of preferred items
- Obsession and Compulsion Recording Template (Chapter 2, Appendix B)
- Operational Definition and Interference Handout (Chapter 2, Appendix C)
- Cheeky Chance materials, one die
- Activities/food items for break/snack
- Reinforcer Checklist (Chapter 1, Appendix B)
- ABC Narrative Form (Chapter 3, Appendix B)
- Examples of Fear Thermometers
- The OCB Cycle Caregiver Handout (Appendix E)

Session Outline

- Homework Review (15 Min.)
- Talking About Obsessions (15 Min.)
- Social Skills Activity: Cheeky Chance (10 Min.)
- Roles and Supports (10 Min.)
- Taking Charge of OCB (20 Min.)
- Break and Snack (10 Min.)
- Designing a Fear Thermometer (15 Min.)
- Assigning Behaviors to Appropriate Zones on My Stimulus Map (15 Min.)
- Assigning Homework (5 Min.)
- Token Exchange and Goodbyes (5 Min.)
- Caregiver Module 2: The OCB Cycle (25 Min.) – To take place during Break and Snack, and Designing a Fear Thermometer

DOI: 10.4324/9781003410126-7

Pre-Session Checklist

• Based on what worked in Session 1, arrange the environment as you feel appropriate.
• You may continue to outline the session activities on a whiteboard or flipchart and check each one off as the session progresses.
• Have child token sheets ready with target prosocial behaviors written on them. Use tokens (e.g., pictures or stickers) that depict each child's interests.

Session Implementation

Homework Review

Use the first few minutes to collect **Caregiver Weekly Data Forms** (Chapter 2, Appendix E) from the previous week. Encourage everyone to greet one another. Ask if anyone would like to share anything about their past week or details about themselves.

Hand out **Token Boards** (Session 1, Appendix A). Remind the children that if they earn all their tokens, this can be exchanged for a mystery prize at the end of the session. Ensure that prosocial behaviors are individualized to each child and are written on each child's token sheet. When you deliver tokens, use behavior-specific praise (e.g., *"I really liked how you asked Quinn how his day was"*).

Briefly review **Caregiver Weekly Data Forms** (Chapter 2, Appendix E) to get an idea of the behaviors that the children have some control over and others that remain difficult. Use these sheets to guide today's exercises. You are collecting information to determine the first obsessive-compulsive behavior (OCB) to address in Session 3 and want to gather information from discussion and observations. Overall, you want to assess the extent to which OCBs are interfering in each child's life. Interference and quality of life will be discussed further in Session 5.

Have children complete the fill-in-the-blank and true-false questions from the workbook activity titled **Homework Review**. If they are unsure of their answers, encourage them to look back at Session 1. Have children share their responses if they feel comfortable and if time permits. Provide them with feedback as needed.

Next, refer to their homework from Session 1. Encourage the child (with the caregiver) to share a few things that they wrote down in completing the **Do-Think-Feel** exercise. This includes the nasty nickname and externalizing activities of what they can say to OCB when it comes around or a picture of OCB. Discuss their compulsions, thoughts (if present), and the identification of parts of the body that may feel "funny" or "weird" before a compulsion is completed. Some children may leave this part blank and that is OK.

Talking About Obsessions

Flip the workbook to the page on **Obsessions**. Tell the group that "O" stands for Obsessions. Explain that *obsession is another word for worries, pictures in your head, or unpleasant or "icky" feelings that you might have.* Adjust wording as needed to fit the developmental needs and maturity of the children (see Psychoeducation and Stimulus Mapping in Chapter 1 for more information). Explain to the group that obsessions often result in performing compulsions (i.e., you may do your compulsion to try to get rid of your worries). Children may not always be able to articulate obsessions. For children who cannot articulate obsessions, or perhaps some of them, remind them that this is perfectly fine. You could explain that sometimes this is hard for people, or it is uncomfortable to talk about. But if they pop into your head today or as you continue to meet, you would like to hear about them.

Simply put, covert behavior is tricky. Go over the examples of obsessions (with accompanying pictures). Children (often with the assistance of caregivers) may point out that they have the same or similar thoughts. Encourage expansion in conversation as appropriate.

Visit the case example of Johnny. Read the case example and have children/caregivers participate as appropriate. Explain that obsessions often cause people to become worried or not feel right. This is just OCB talking. Then, a person might do something like wash their hands over and over again until they feel that the germs are gone. This is OCB sending incorrect messages to Johnny again. Consider the developmental and cognitive profiles of each child when explaining.

Using the workbook as a guide, ask the children what Johnny could say or do to OCB when he starts to get worried (instead of washing his hands over and over). Generate loose discussion and involve caregivers (e.g., *"Does Johnny need to wash his hands many, many times? OCB just told him his hands are germy, but even if they were, was there a need to wash them over and over or would washing them once be OK?"*). Explain again that OCB can be tricky, and we need to become aware of this character to outsmart or beat it!

In identifying their obsessions, have children refer back to Session 1 of their workbook where they wrote down or drew pictures of a few compulsions. Ask them to write out at least two worries or unpleasant feelings that they might have before doing the compulsions in the **Obsessions** section of the workbook. Ensure you have the **Obsession and Compulsion Recording Template** (Chapter 2, Appendix B) and the **Operational Definitions and Interference Handout** (Chapter 2, Appendix C) from the assessment available. Attempt to have children think of obsessions on their own but use the assessment sheet as needed to fill in the blanks. Children are likely not going to be able to remember all compulsions and obsessions.

For those who have identified limited obsessions, continue to probe what they think about right before engaging in compulsions, and/or ask why they need to perform compulsions (see Table 2.3 in Chapter 2 for suggestions for probing for information regarding compulsions and obsessions). Try not to lead them in any way (e.g., "Do you wash your hands because you're worried about getting sick?"). They may accept an obsession you give them for many reasons, including escaping from a difficult or uncomfortable task. If the child does not verbalize obsessions, focus on reviewing compulsions. Assist the caregiver/child dyads as necessary.

Encourage children to share their acknowledged compulsions (and obsessions) with their group members. If there are commonalities between group members, you may comment on this. Provide behavior-specific praise and tokens for completing the exercise and/or sharing their thoughts.

At this stage and as the sessions progress, you may obtain more information about obsessions and additional operant functions. You may also attempt to gain more information about antecedents, establishing operations, setting events, and additional functions beyond anxiety (see Chapter 3 for an overview of functions). This will be helpful when conducting your functional behavior assessment (FBA) and designing the multicomponent intervention for the child's first targeted OCB for Session 3. Generate some ideas on which OCB should be tackled first using information derived from the clinical assessment, your observations, upcoming exercises, and discussion with the child/caregiver.

Social Skills Activity: Cheeky Chance

Cheeky Chance involves children taking turns rolling a die and choosing an activity to complete based on the number rolled (e.g., if a five is rolled and the child chooses jumping jacks, everyone will do five jumping jacks). This is a beginner social skill activity (see Chapter 4 for further details).

Instructions: Explain that everyone is going to have a chance to roll the die and that the person who rolls gets to decide which activity everyone is going to play. The number on the die is the number of times the activity is played. For example, if a child rolls a six and they want to do jumping jacks, everyone will do six jumping jacks. If needed, demonstrate rolling the die and playing a game before the children take a turn. Both physical and non-physical activities should be encouraged. When the person has finished their turn, encourage everyone to give a high-five to the people next to them. Continue until everyone has had a turn.

In a one-on-one setting, the therapist and/or caregivers can participate in the activity by taking turns rolling the die and performing the actions alongside the child. See Chapter 4 for additional modifications for individual therapy.

Roles and Supports

The **Roles and Supports** activity in the workbook builds on the conversation around the child being the boss. Talk to children about being in charge or the boss of OCB. Ask questions like *"Who likes to be the boss?"* and *"What do you like to be the boss of?"* To do this, first ask the children to draw themselves or write their names at the top of the mountain. Then, let them know that they will not be alone in fighting or bossing back OCB. They will have many helpers to cheer them on and support them while they take on the OCB challenge. Have them write down or draw their chosen helpers (e.g., family, friends, pets, and therapists). If they have characters that are special to them, encourage them to draw them as well. Refer to Chapter 1, Psychoeducation and Stimulus Mapping for a case example of Sadie and a picture she independently drew of herself and her support team.

Taking Charge of OCB

Have children work individually (with caregiver assistance). If administering group therapy, you may move caregiver/child dyads to different parts of the room or separate tables. This will aid in decreasing distractions and increase attention to the task. Children will be discussing private issues and may not want others to overhear.

The goal of the **Taking Charge of OCB** workbook exercise is for the child, with the assistance of their caregivers, the **Obsession and**

Compulsion Recording Template (Chapter 2, Appendix B) and the **Operational Definitions and Interference Handout** (Chapter 2, Appendix C), to write out compulsions (and associated obsessions) that will be addressed in treatment. Encourage children to take as much of an active role as they feel comfortable. Use information from the clinical assessment to support the child in completing this exercise. Probe obsessions as you see fit and build on previous exercises with obsessions (see Table 2.3 from Chapter 2 for examples of probes).

At this point, you may begin the discussion of which OCB should be tackled first. Ideally, it would be one in which the child can resist performing the compulsion, at least some of the time. This can also be talked about further with the **Mapping OCB** exercise (see below). You don't want to begin with an extremely difficult OCB as this may discourage the child.

You can refer back to the **Obsessions** activity where they wrote out or drew two compulsions (and obsessions, if present). You are gradually shaping their behavior and the amount of information that they provide or write down. They can copy what they wrote in this activity so that they have the first two obsessions and compulsions complete.

Note: At this point, children will complete Break and Snack (10 Min.) and Designing a Fear Thermometer (15 Min.) while caregivers complete Caregiver Module 2: The OCB Cycle (25 Min.).

Break and Snack

You may continue to offer snacks from the **Reinforcer Checklist** (Chapter 1, Appendix B). Depending on your policies, snacks may be prepared ahead of time or caregivers may be asked to bring in snacks.

Allow this break period to be child-directed (e.g., a child may want to draw or attempt to initiate a game with you). You can capitalize on this time to build rapport with the children or facilitate rapport building within the group. If helpful, use a timer and give children reminders of the time remaining.

You may use this time to observe OCBs or contrive situations to collect descriptive data (if possible) using the **ABC Narrative Form** (Chapter 3, Appendix B) or you may use one of your own.

Designing a Fear Thermometer

It may be difficult for children to identify the varying intensity of their anxiety. Your goal with the **Fear Thermometer** workbook activity is to help them understand that anxiety or unpleasant feelings do not simply turn on and off. They gradually increase, like the temperature rising on a thermometer. Show examples of different ways to design fear thermometers (e.g., red zone, yellow zone, green zone; a number scale or no number scale). You want them to be able to differentiate between distressed/anxious (higher number or level) and calm (lower number or level).

Some children may benefit from emotion recognition training (see Emotion Recognition Training in Chapter 1). For example, emotion cards can be paired with parts of the fear thermometer to help children recognize which emotions best fit each zone, such as relaxed in the green zone, nervous in the yellow zone, and terrified in the red zone. Then, let the children add to the drawing of the fear thermometer. They can also draw their own fear rater on the blank page if they prefer. Use concrete examples of non-OCB experiences to help them anchor their scale. Start with a non-OCB example to rate the intensity (e.g., a scary movie or talking about being up high on playground equipment or an amusement ride). Try to find something to anchor the lowest point of the scale. Ask probing questions about how they feel around that stimulus or situation (e.g., *How does your body feel when you are in the green zone?*). Then try and find something to anchor the higher points of the scale. When each child is done designing the thermometer, do a quick check to make sure they understand how it is used.

Let them know that they are going to use their fear thermometer or fear rater to rate their fears or let us know how distressed they would feel if they could not engage in their compulsions. Using miniature sticky notes, have the children write down at least three to five of their compulsions (and obsessions, if they can) from the list they completed in the previous section on **Taking Charge of OCB**. Then, have them use their fear thermometer to rate how upset they would feel if they couldn't do their compulsions.

Assigning Behaviors to Appropriate Zones on My Stimulus Map

Next, review the three **Mapping OCB** zones (OCB Zone, OCB/ME Zone, and ME Zone). You are going to have the child map at least three to five OCBs by sticking them onto one of the zones. The OCB Zone is where the child has no control over the behavior and OCB always wins. The OCB/ME Zone is where the child has some control over the behavior (or resistance in performing the compulsion), and the ME Zone is where the child has complete control. Ensure the children understand the three zones before placing the miniature sticky notes with compulsions on them. Encourage children to use their fear ratings to guide where the sticky notes go. For example, if their rating is a 4, it may be placed in the OCB/Me Zone; whereas, if their rating is an 8, it would be placed in the OCB Zone. At this point, not many behaviors will be in the ME Zone.

Some of the OCBs should be behaviors that children may have some control over and, therefore, may be possible targets over the next few weeks. You may not have the chance to map all OCBs. Focus on behaviors where the child seems to have the most control and the OCBs they choose to add.

Stimulus mapping will likely be continued at the beginning of Session 3. This is when you will discuss the first OCB that will be tackled.

Assigning Homework

Assign homework to the children. Go over the **OCB News** section of the workbook. Have caregivers assist their children in answering the wh-questions for the first OCB they will tackle next session. Encourage children to complete this before the next session and use their fear thermometer or rater to rate how they would feel if they weren't allowed to do the compulsion.

Token Exchange and Goodbyes

Complete the token exchange where tokens are exchanged for a grab bag item of their choosing. Encourage them to say goodbye to one another (if run in a group format). Just like in Session 1, this may need to be modeled and prompted.

Caregiver Module 2: The OCB Cycle

Review and Introduction

Distribute new caregiver data sheets (see Chapter 2, Appendix E). Let caregivers know to bring forward issues or challenges when tackling OCBs, or any new OCBs that arise.

Tell the caregivers that this week's module will focus on the **OCB Cycle** (Appendix E).

Box 7.1   Behavioral Skills Training

Each caregiver module is structured using the four-step behavioral skills training model. As described in Chapter 1 (Weekly Caregiver Coaching Modules: Scaffolding of Treatment Components), this empirically supported model is used to teach individuals new skills by following four steps: instructions, modeling, rehearsal, and feedback.

The behavioral skills training model can be modified to meet each caregiver's individual needs. For example:

- **Instructions** can be modified to be more of a discussion than a didactic lecture;
- **Modeling** can occur with frequent breaks in which you explain what you are modeling and why;
- **Rehearsal** might not occur in session if the caregiver is not comfortable with demonstrating the skill in front of others (e.g., the caregiver can rehearse the skill with a family member at home) or needs additional time to process the instructions given; and
- **Feedback** should be tailored to each caregiver's preference (e.g., verbal vs. written; in the moment vs. after rehearsal has taken place).

These steps can be repeated until the caregiver is proficient and feels confident in performing the new skill. Any of the steps can be combined (e.g., modeling and rehearsal) or prompts can be added. By adapting the process to meet each caregiver's needs, you can develop and maintain rapport, reduce the caregiver's anxiety, and maximize the caregiver's learning benefits.

Instruction

Give each caregiver a blank copy of the **OCB Cycle** (Appendix E) and explain it using caregiver-friendly language:

- Obsessions are unwanted or intrusive thoughts (e.g., "My hands are contaminated") that cause children distress, anxiety, and/or negative physiological sensations (e.g., racing heart rate or rapid breathing).

- To get rid of these unpleasant sensations, children engage in compulsions (e.g., excessive handwashing).
- The child experiences temporary relief from these unpleasant sensations; however, when their distress arises again, the cycle repeats.

Explain that compulsions may occur even in the absence of obsessions. Perhaps there isn't a thought (like in the case where the function is sensory reinforcement) but engaging in the compulsion makes the child feel 'just right' or experience positive sensory stimulation (e.g., the visual of aligning objects in a certain way). It is also possible that the child may not know what obsessions or thoughts they are experiencing or have difficulty expressing these thoughts due to limited introspection. Compulsions may still occur to alleviate distress or anxiety.

Furthermore, sometimes it's unclear how these compulsions developed and sometimes they happen at random. For instance, a child might engage in a random behavior and that behavior happened to help alleviate their distress. From that point forward, the child may continue to engage in that behavior when they experience distress unless someone helps them find an alternative way to manage their distress. You can let the caregivers know they will learn more about this in future sessions and modules.

Modeling

Show the caregiver how to fill out the **OCB Cycle** using a simple example, such as thoughts of contamination or worries about someone getting hurt (obsession) leading to repetitive handwashing or arranging stuffed animals (compulsion) to temporarily alleviate thoughts/distress. See Chapter 1, (Obsessive-Compulsive Behaviors and Perceived Operant Functions) for additional examples.

Helpful hint! If completing this module in a group, this can be modeled on a whiteboard or chalkboard. If completing it individually, this can be done using a therapist's copy of the handout.

Rehearsal

Support the caregiver in filling out the **OCB Cycle** using one of their child's compulsions and obsessions (if present). If needed, you can help the caregiver come up with ideas. Use your best judgment to gauge each caregiver's level of knowledge and support required.

If rehearsal isn't possible, tell the caregiver that this will be reviewed thoroughly during individual programming for OCBs later in the session.

Feedback

Provide positive and specific praise when the caregiver completes either a component of or the full cycle correctly (e.g., "That's right. You identified your child's compulsion perfectly.") and corrective feedback for incorrect/incomplete components (e.g., "Not quite. Try this instead.").

Box 7.2   Tentative Caregivers

Some caregivers have difficulty practicing skills in front of others. Encourage caregivers by letting them know it might feel awkward at first, but as we become familiar with the skill, it will become second nature. Appropriate reinforcement from the therapist is important in reducing performance anxiety. If the caregiver is still reluctant, rehearsal can take place individually or even at home. Emphasize that, regardless, practicing skills is an important part of the intervention process and will help their child be successful.

Scheduling Follow-Up Meetings

Take a few minutes to schedule phone calls with caregivers to complete any outstanding FBAs. Look at Chapter 3 for a detailed explanation of this process. If you did not explain the process to the caregiver in Session 1, let them know you will be calling them to discuss their child's compulsion(s) and why they may be engaging in them. This will involve asking a series of questions about the behavior. This appointment can take place over the telephone, virtually, or in person and will take approximately 30 minutes (this time can be divided into two shorter sessions if preferred by the caregiver). Lastly, remind caregivers when direct observations will occur (at home or in the clinic). You may have completed direct observations during the clinical assessment but additional observations (e.g., during snack or other activities in Session 1) are always helpful.

Additional Therapist Preparation for Session 3

- Complete planning using the **Cognitive Behavioral Skills Template** (Appendix A). See Chapter 1 for a thorough explanation of each of the strategies.

- Complete the indirect FBA for the first OCB to be targeted during exposure via telephone, videoconference, or in person, using the guidance in Chapter 3.
- Combine the results of the indirect assessment and your data from direct observations.
- Fill out the **Competing Behavior Model** (Appendix B) with the information you have gathered and complete the **Functional Behavior Assessment and Intervention (FBAI) Summary Form** (Appendix C). A sample completed form is in Appendix D. See Chapter 3 for the full walk-through of the FBA process.

Appendix A

Cognitive Behavioral Skills Template

OCBs	Bossing Back Statements/ Actions	Cultivating Nonattachment and Coping Strategies	Other Things I Need or Like	Thinking Differently and Self-Talk Related to OCB	E/RP Sheet Preparation
	Examples: Bossing statements; doing karate	*Examples:* Breathing or sitting with OCB	Have the FBAI sheet ready	*Example:* Cognitive Restructuring and/or potential self-statements	Review all components on the Stepping It Up Worksheet

1. Compulsion:

   Obsession:

2. Compulsion:

   Obsession:

3. Compulsion:

   Obsession:

4. Compulsion:

   Obsession:

5. Compulsion:

   Obsession:

To assist you in filling out the template, you have the following resources:

- Three sample completed **Stepping It Up** worksheets (see Children's Workbook and Session 3).
- Table 1.1 in Chapter 1 offers several examples of behaviors, including the starting point and desired level for each OCB.

Appendix B

Competing Behavior Model

See the competing behavior model in Chapter 3 for more detailed instructions which will inform the FBAI Summary Form (see next page on the FBAI that you give to the caregiver).

Name: _____ Date: _____ OCB: _____

What events affect the likelihood of the antecedent resulting in an OCB?	What events or stimuli reliably result in the OCB? What seems to trigger the behavior?	What does the OCB look like?		What is the likely function of this behavior?
Establishing Operation(s)	**Antecedent(s)**	**OCB(s)**	**Maintaining Consequence(s)**	**Function(s)**

	Replacement Behavior	

Establishing Operation Strategies	**Antecedent Strategies**	**Teaching Strategies**	**Consequence Strategies**

Appendix C

Functional Behavior Assessment and Intervention (FBAI) Summary Form

See the competing behavior model in Chapter 3 for instructions. Fill out the form for the first OCB.

OCB(s) Compulsion/Obsession	Likely Function(s) Why the OCB happens	Function-based Intervention(s) How to reduce the OCB(s) *Implement during exposure or after gradual exposure step
1.	1.	1.
2.	2.	2.
3.	3.	3.
4.	4.	4.
5.	5.	5.

Appendix D

Sample of Completed Functional Behavior Assessment and Intervention (FBAI) Summary Form

OCB(s) *Compulsion/ Obsession*	Likely Function(s) *Why the OCB happens*	Function-based Intervention(s) *How to reduce the OCB(s) *Implement during exposure or after gradual exposure step*
Compulsion: Repetitive handwashing (Obsession: Thoughts of contamination)	Escape from anxiety	**Escape from anxiety**: Redirect to coping skills (e.g., deep breathing after 3 minutes of handwashing instead of 10 minutes (baseline), or encourage positive self-statements during gradual exposure or after it is completed.
	Access to attention	**Access to attention:** Minimize attention for OCB during and after gradual exposure and provide lots of attention for engaging in conversation about a preferred topic unrelated to the OCB. This may include discussion of coping strategies.
Compulsion: Arranging stuffed animals (Obsession: "Not just right" feeling in body)	Escape from anxiety	**Escape from anxiety**: Redirect to coping skills (e.g., counting or bossing back statements) during gradual exposure or after it is completed.
	Access to sensory stimulation (enjoying the look of the arrangement)	**Access to sensory stimulation:** Provide access to a select number of sensory toys to arrange during the day.

Appendix E

The OCB Cycle Caregiver Handout

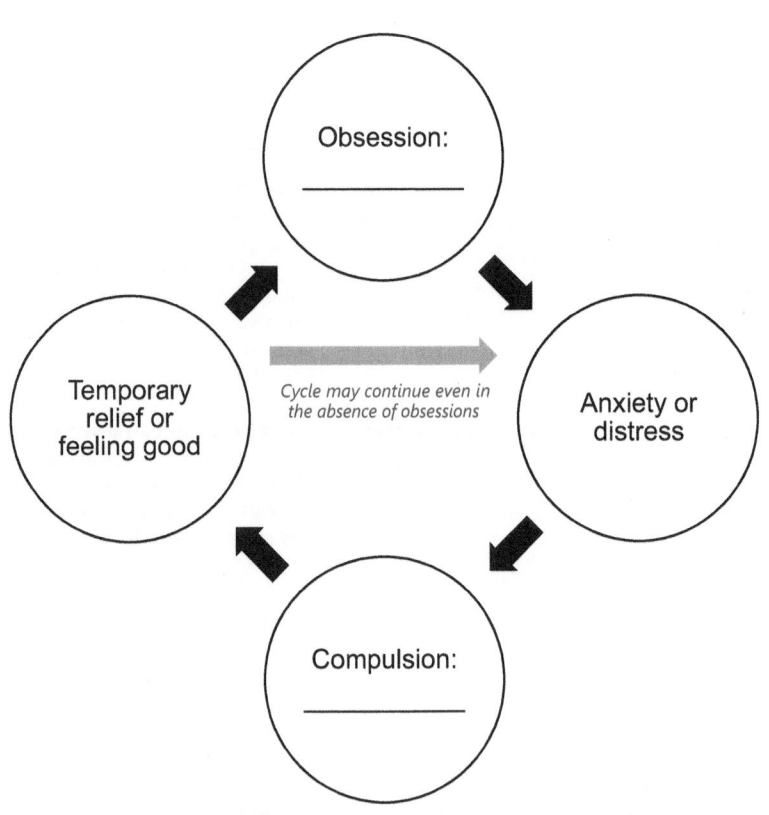

Chapter 8

Session 3
CBT Skills Training and Beginning E/RP for First OCB

Materials

- Children's Workbook
- Flipchart/Whiteboard
- Caregiver Weekly Data Form (Chapter 2, Appendix E)
- Token Board (Session 1, Appendix A)
- Tokens and grab bag of preferred items
- Miniature sticky notes for the OCB Stimulus Map
- Fear thermometer
- Obsession and Compulsion Recording Template (Chapter 2, Appendix B)
- Operational Definitions and Interference Form (Chapter 2, Appendix C)
- Activities/food items for break/snack
- ABC Narrative Form (Chapter 3, Appendix B)
- Reinforcer Checklist (Chapter 1, Appendix B)
- Collect, Pass, Run, and Sort – The Running Relay materials: three sheets of paper, four labeled plastic baskets, three bags, and three sets of grocery item pictures
- Cognitive Behavioral Skills Template (Session 2, Appendix A)

Session Outline

- Homework Review (15 Min.)
- Revisit the OCB Map (15 Min.)
- CBT Skills Training and Designing an Individualized Treatment Plan for the First OCB (20 Min.)
- Break and Snack (10 Min.)
- Social Skills Activity: Collect, Pass, Run and Sort – The Running Relay (15 Min.)
- Programming for First OCB: Continue to Introduce Treatment Components and Complete the E/RP Worksheet (20 Min.)
- Individualized Intervention for OCB #1 and Homework (20 Min.)

DOI: 10.4324/9781003410126-8

- Token Exchange and Goodbyes (5 Min.)
- Caregiver Module 3: Introduction to Functional Behavior Assessment and FBAI (25 Min.) - To take place during Break and Snack, and Collect, Pass, Run, and Sort – The Running Relay

Pre-Session Checklist

- Arrange the environment (e.g., seating) as you feel appropriate.
- You may continue to outline the session activities on a whiteboard or flipchart.
- Have child **Token Boards** ready with prosocial behaviors written on them. Vary tokens to depict preferred pictures or stickers to maintain interest.
- Complete the **Cognitive Behavioral Skills Template** (Session 2, Appendix A) for the first OCB.
- Prepare new **Caregiver Weekly Data Forms** (Chapter 2, Appendix E).
- Complete the **Functional Behavior Assessment and Intervention (FBAI) Summary Form** (based on functional behavior assessment completed) (Session 2, Appendix C).

Session Implementation

Homework Review

Use the first few minutes to collect **Caregiver Weekly Data Forms** (Chapter 2, Appendix E) from the previous week. Review the session outline on the whiteboard that roughly matches the schedule in the Children's Workbook. Children will likely attend to the session outline automatically as they familiarize themselves with the routine. Hand out the **Token Boards** (Session 1, Appendix A) with prosocial behaviors written on them for today's session. As sessions progress, you may modify the list of prosocial behaviors.

Remind children that if they earn their ten tokens, this can be exchanged for a prize at the end of the session. When you deliver tokens for target prosocial behaviors, use behavior-specific praise. Older children or more developmentally mature children may choose to self-monitor their behavior or derive their own method.

Strengths

Have the children state at least one of their strengths or say something that they are proud of. Review material from the previous session on believing in themselves.

Have children talk about their **OCB News** for the first obsessive-compulsive behavior (OCB) they completed as homework for Session 2. Caregivers can provide as much assistance as needed. This will likely be the behavior that you program for today, and the child (with their support team) will tackle it over the next week. Reviewing the **OCB News** will allow you to get an idea of the child's awareness of this OCB and knowledge of the "WH" questions as well as setting events and antecedents. As part of this exercise, review thermometer ratings if appropriate.

Revisit the OCB Map

Review the **Mapping OCB** activity from Session 2 and have children finish writing compulsions (and talking about obsessions where appropriate). Refer to the **Obsession and Compulsion Recording Template** (Chapter 2, Appendix B). It is good to have children flipping back and forth in the workbook as we want to familiarize them with it, and our hope is that they will refer to it post-treatment. Like the last session, have the child write their compulsions on miniature sticky notes. Do the thermometer ratings for each compulsion and add the ratings to the sticky notes. Then, have the child place the compulsions on the **Mapping OCB** worksheet. Using the stimulus map and the **Caregiver Weekly Data Forms** (Chapter 2, Appendix E), comment on the targeted OCB for this session. Also, this is a great opportunity to discuss possible OCBs that continue to be interfering, supported by the **Operational Definitions and Interference Form** (Chapter 2, Appendix C), and that are possible targets for Session 4. Try to consider OCBs where children can sometimes resist them or the urge to do the compulsion. This can also be discussed in Caregiver Module 3 when scheduling the functional behavior assessment (FBA).

CBT Skills Training and Designing an Individualized Treatment Plan for the First OCB

Have the **Cognitive Behavioral Skills Template** (Session 2, Appendix A) and the **Functional Behavior Assessment and Intervention (FBAI) Summary Form** (Session 2, Appendix C) completed as preparation for this session. When programming for the first OCB, you may want to refer to Chapter 1 for a more thorough explanation of each of the cognitive behavioral therapy (CBT) strategies and Chapter 3 for the full walk-through of the functional behavior assessment process.

Review the cognitive behavioral skills components to co-design the child's first OCB treatment plan with the child and caregiver. For the first

OCB, to prevent fatigue and maintain the child's motivation, we find it helpful to review the different cognitive techniques and CBT skills in pieces (with accompanying visuals from the workbook to help children stay engaged and take part in hands-on activities). This often can be challenging for the first OCB but usually becomes easier as you and the child (with the assistance of their support team) learn what strategies are preferred, and if they prefer to continue using the same strategies or explore new ones.

Believing in Myself: What I Can Do and Say to OCB

Children and youth who are aware of their obsessions and compulsions may have a learned history of self-blame regarding not being able to resist the urge to engage in compulsions. Through psychoeducation and the exercises in the sessions thus far (e.g., **The OCB Story** in Session 1 about OCB's incorrect message of the need to take a long shower), we explain to the child that their brain may be sending out incorrect messages, but this is just OCB talking. These messages do not require immediate attention and, thus, engagement in the compulsion. Refer to the sections in Chapter 1 on Psychoeducation and Stimulus Mapping for a more in-depth discussion of psychoeducation.

Beginning in Session 1, we teach children to externalize OCBs and let them just come and go. In Sessions 1 and 2, children were taught to tell OCB to go away; for example, "Beat it!" or simply acknowledge OCB's presence (e.g., "Hi there, OCB" [nickname]). You are teaching the child to either boss back OCB or accept OCB's presence, and if left long enough, OCB will just go away (like the pins and needles example in Session 1).

For the first OCB, you will begin with the workbook activity of **Believing in Myself: What I Can Do and Say to OCB**. It is best to begin here as this is something the children are likely familiar with (given exposure to bossing back statements in Sessions 1 and 2) and may require minimal response effort given they have already generated responses (which they can be prompted to refer to). For this exercise, they can write out statements or have a caregiver scribe their responses. For different types of responses, see preferred modalities in Chapter 1, ASD Adaptations Embedded into Fb-CBT. Encourage children to read sample responses (e.g., "Beat it!") and add to them or generate responses of their own and write in the thought bubbles.

Note that they can also write things they can "do" to OCB such as "I'm going to beat you up, OCB!" or "Here's a karate move for you!"

and demonstrate the movement. We have had children demonstrate karate moves in session! Be mindful that there are several treatment components, and OCB #1 is only the beginning to familiarize them with this. Given time constraints, it is OK to have them generate a few responses and then move on to the next technique. As sessions progress, they will become increasingly fluent in using the techniques and will become more independent in choosing what works for them.

My Toolbox

You may now begin to add techniques to the child's toolbox. The **My Toolbox** activity in the workbook shows a list of coping techniques (with pictures) that a child or youth may choose to do when the urge to engage in the compulsion arises. First, read aloud or have the child read the text in the image of the Children's Workbook. When introducing the toolbox and selected techniques, observe what the child gravitates to. Also, ask the child if any coping techniques have worked for them in the past and if they would like to use them for the first OCB. There are blank boxes to write in techniques or draw pictures. Be mindful of time constraints and response effort on the part of the child. Choose one or two techniques to focus on for the first OCB.

Have them practice the technique and place a checkmark in the box after attempting it. Model the technique and provide prompting as needed. You may need to teach and model how to engage in a particular coping strategy, or children may be familiar and need less demonstration on how to engage in them.

Between sessions, the caregiver may also need to model the technique or provide prompting at home. The caregiver may need to give verbal prompts, but to minimize prompt dependency, you could encourage the caregiver to write out the techniques or have them handy on a device (e.g., an iPad). The general idea is that, over time, children will become more independent in implementing treatment strategies (e.g., independently initiating a breathing exercise when they are starting to feel anxious), and the caregiver will gradually fade out their assistance.

Ensure you remind the caregiver to deliver praise specific to the coping strategy. We want them to be acknowledged for their hard work. For some caregivers, this will come naturally, and others may need prompting from you. Importantly, they need to be encouraged to both practice techniques but also use them in real-life situations.

Encourage children to practice techniques throughout the day. Intermittent practice may also contribute to children remaining regulated or in a relaxed state throughout the day.

You will get feedback from the child on the chosen techniques next session and can continue to explore others as the sessions progress. The idea is to develop fluency in using the techniques in their toolbox when needed and to expose the child or youth to a wide range of options that they can use now and when therapy ends.

When discussing homework for this session (**Stepping It Up: Completing My Exposures**), they will write three techniques that they would like to practice and use during exposures. When beginning the Exposure/Response Prevention (E/RP) phase with daily exposures for their first goal (or OCB to tackle), the child will hopefully be successful at completing their daily goal (e.g., five minutes of handwashing with the original duration being ten minutes) and then engage in a chosen strategy (instead of completing the full compulsion). Children will often talk about feeling anxious or not "just right". They may also describe emotions like anger or frustration, or you may see overt indicators of distress (e.g., facial changes, rubbing/pulling hair). The chosen strategy (e.g., deep breathing) will act as a replacement behavior for the full compulsion (e.g., 10 min of handwashing) and help in alleviating the anxiety and/or distracting them.

Box 8.1 Reminder!

Remember to give behavior-specific praise and deliver tokens as appropriate throughout the session.

Note: At this point, children will complete Break and Snack (10 Min.) and Social Skills Activity: Collect, Pass, Run, and Sort – The Running Relay (15 Min.) while caregivers complete Caregiver Module 3 (25 Min.).

Break and Snack

You may continue to offer snacks from the **Reinforcer Checklist** (Chapter 1, Appendix B). Depending on your policies, snacks may be prepared ahead of time, or caregivers may be asked to bring in snacks.

Allow this break period to be child-directed (e.g., a child may want to draw or attempt to initiate a game with you). You can capitalize on this time to build rapport with the children or facilitate rapport building within the group. If helpful, use a timer and give children reminders of the time remaining.

You may use this time to observe OCBs or contrive situations to collect descriptive data (if possible) using the **ABC Narrative Form** (Chapter 3, Appendix B), or you may use one of your own.

Social Skills Activity: Collect, Pass, Run, and Sort – The Running Relay

The Collect, Pass, Run, and Sort – Running Relay involves children working together to complete a relay and scavenger hunt. This is an intermediate social skill activity (see Chapter 4 for further details).

Instructions: Place grocery item pictures around the room and mark the floor with prompts for where each child should stand according to their role (e.g., Passer, Runner, Sorter). Each picture corresponds with a corresponding picture in each child's grocery basket. In group therapy, inform the children to get into groups of three and assign each child one of the three roles. Inform the children that the goal is to collect all the grocery items as a team using their designated roles. If needed, you can model the scavenger hunt. Say *"On your mark, get set, GO!"* to start the race. Prompt the children to encourage one another. Once all items have been retrieved and sorted, have the children switch roles and repeat the activity. If time permits, do this until each child has had a turn playing each of the three roles.

In a one-on-one setting, the therapist and caregiver may participate in the relay race with the child, or the child can perform the relay more than once and try to do it in the fastest time. See Chapter 4 for additional modifications.

Programming for First OCB: Continue to Introduce Treatment Components and Complete the E/RP Worksheet

Other Things I Need or Like

The **Other Things I Need or Like** workbook activity supports identifying functional replacement behaviors for OCB. Have the child turn to the appropriate page in the Children's Workbook. Explain that these are more techniques they can choose. Have the caregiver refer to the **Functional Behavior Assessment and Intervention (FBAI) Summary Form** (Session 3, Appendix C), likely functions, and potential techniques that they were just provided during the Caregiver Module. You can have the caregiver take the lead on some parts if they are comfortable. For example, if access to attention from the caregiver was identified as a likely function, you can assist the caregiver in talking with the child about having more conversations or engaging in social activities when they feel the urge to perform the compulsion. These techniques may need to be written down in the Children's Workbook (e.g., brainstorming types of conversations) along with when the child should use them.

In Chapters 1 and 2, we discussed a youth (Jess) who had a fear that his food would not be digested and repeatedly asked for reassurance from his caregiver. Asking for and receiving repetitive reassurance was the compulsion and lessened the youth's anxiety. As a team, you and the caregiver can talk about the child liking social attention (similar to many of us) but that social attention and conversation can be accomplished in many ways. In the case of Jess, it was discussing sports statistics and then interspersing less preferred topics.

Suppose access to attention did arise as a perceived function during the functional behavior assessment. In that case, a replacement such as having a back-and-forth conversation may need to be explicitly taught by breaking the skill into smaller components. Functional communication training (FCT) may also be used. Chapter 3 provides a definition and examples of FCT. The workbook also includes examples of other functional replacement behaviors, like taking a break or engaging with sensory items, that address functions other than access to attention.

Thinking Differently and Outsmarting My OCB

The **Thinking Differently and Outsmarting My OCB** activity is the final set of cognitive and behavioral skills. You need to use your discretion as to how much time you spend on this activity. See Chapter 1, Thinking Differently: Cognitive Restructuring for a more detailed description of cognitive restructuring and self-talk. Many school-age children have a difficult time articulating the obsessions or thoughts and physiological sensations that precede compulsions. If children in your group experience this, you may spend minimal time on this section and move to the part of the worksheet on **Outsmarting my OCB.**

In Chapter 1, we discuss probability and personal responsibility; these concepts need to be individualized to children. We go over several examples that you may choose to refer to when programming for each child. With these concepts, you are working on "disproving OCB" and challenging faulty assumptions. If the child is aware of the obsession and views it as unreasonable you can work on the faulty connection between the obsession and compulsion. It is possible that this may motivate the child to use their chosen techniques and resist the urge to engage in the compulsion. For example, Molly from Chapter 1 needed to slam the door three times to get rid of the tension in her hand. By reviewing that OCB often sends out incorrect messages and challenging the belief that slamming the door multiple times would lessen the uncomfortable feeling in her hand, we were able to engage in cognitive restructuring about the irrationality of the compulsion. Teaching the child that these feelings will come and go (like pins and needles) or perhaps this is just OCB talking may break the connection.

You may attempt to restructure or reframe thoughts if appropriate and the child's cognitive and developmental profile allows for it. For example, a child may be afraid that they will get sick and die after someone sneezes. You could challenge this from many different angles. You could look at probability (in simple terms; perhaps look at the primary reasons people get sick and the chances of getting ill if someone sneezes on you). In this case, you are getting at the child's overestimation of feared consequences (in the case of a sneeze).

Regarding fears of contamination, we have found it helpful with some kids to engage in education around the subject matter. In the case of germs, they are present everywhere. How about the fact that exposure to germs may help to train your immune system? Refer to the case in Chapter 1 of Sadie and the use of knowledge and facts to disprove OCB. Challenging the thoughts, obsessions, or images may also be accomplished with visuals and vocal explanation (perhaps in the form of social stories) and checking out facts and knowledge via the internet or books. Be creative and adapt to the child's cognitive profile and general learning style.

When completing the worksheet on **Thinking Differently about OCB**, you may have the child write out key statements from your discussions. For some children, this may be helpful.

For children who do not have a thought or perhaps have a partial thought, you may move to the personalized self-talk statements or **Outsmarting My OCB.** The difference between these statements and externalizing statements is that they are statements or rules specific to the targeted OCB. They may be statements building from knowledge learned in cognitive restructuring, or they may be rules that the child follows that are specific to the OCB (e.g., "I've learned my teeth will be clean if I brush for 3 minutes!"). Last, you may explore replacing negative self-statements with positive self-statements. For example, a child may say "I have to check the door five times. I can't stop." The "I can't" may be a theme for many OCBs. You may try to replace this with "I can do it. I'm not going to let OCB beat me" OR "I'm just going to check three times. I'm on my way to outsmarting OCB!"

Rewarding Yourself

Have the child turn to the **Rewarding Yourself** activities in the workbook. Read the text aloud or have the child and/or caregiver do so. Explain that "saying no to OCB" or resisting the urge to do a compulsion can be hard. Say something like, *it's time to write down some rewards you can work for when completing your exposures, and say no to OCB!* Explain to children that they will write daily rewards on their homework sheet to earn when they're being brave and bossing back OCB. Try to make the connection for them between the rewards and completing their exposures (and using their coping techniques) each day.

If they need assistance, have their **Reinforcer Checklist** (see Chapter 1, Appendix B) handy. Preferences do change frequently for some children and youth, so it can be helpful to readminister it. In our experience, children are often good at generating tangible rewards based on things they engage in daily (e.g., iPad use). Some other examples include spending 15–20 min doing their activity of choice with a caregiver or choosing their favorite meal for dinner. The child does not need to fill out all five rewards. Come up with a few and then move on to the next page. Immediate reinforcement is better than delayed reinforcement. Therefore, children will choose daily rewards for completing exposures. Explain to the caregiver and child that many of the rewards should be small rewards that can be delivered each day. See Chapter 1, Adaptations Embedded into Fb-CBT for more extensive information on this topic.

Small and Big Rewards

Sometimes children have a difficult time separating out small rewards from big rewards. The **Small and Big Rewards** can be used to explore different types of rewards that can be differentially delivered daily versus at the end of the week, or for easier homework tasks compared to more challenging tasks. Big rewards can be given at the end of the week contingent on the child's success throughout the week (and the delivery of daily rewards). Given the focus on small rewards on the **Rewarding Yourself** sheet, you may want to encourage children to copy what they have already generated. If you have generated sufficient information in the **Rewarding Yourself** activity, you may choose to skip this sheet. You can refer to this sheet when completing the **Stepping It Up: Completing My Exposures** homework to identify small rewards for daily practice and large rewards for sustained success.

Individualized Intervention for OCB #1 and Homework

Believing in Myself: Stepping It Up and Completing Exposures!

In the workbook, you will see an example of a completed **Stepping It Up: Completing My Exposures** sheet targeting a handwashing OCB for Jaden. Go over the pieces with the child and caregiver as an example. We suggest beginning with writing out the goal and the daily exposures from bottom to top. In the example, when Jaden began treatment, handwashing occurred for ten minutes. Therapy took place on Tuesday evenings, so the first exposure (or step) was to be completed on Wednesday (seven minutes). In collaboration with Jaden and his caregiver, we agreed to systematically reduce the time to an ending weekly goal of one minute or the desired level (see top step of worksheet). Explain that Jaden wanted to get down to his desired level of handwashing for one minute in one week. In some cases, this may be reasonable, and in other cases, getting a behavior to the terminal goal may take more time. That is perfectly OK and should be emphasized to the child.

You may want to now talk about the fact that bossing back OCB is often hard and talk to the child or youth about using our coping techniques when doing so. Review the coping techniques for handwashing written at the top of the sheet. Discuss that Jaden chose a bossing back statement (Buzz off, OCB!), talking about sports with mom (the child enjoyed talking about sports and it was identified during functional behavior assessment that social attention was a function), and taking deep breaths. At this point, to keep the child engaged, you could ask the child or youth one coping technique they might choose when getting to their OCB.

Explain to the child that now that coping techniques have been discussed, we can move to progress tracking. Emphasize that Jaden attempted to combat OCB gradually (i.e., less and less handwashing), and the goal was to practice three exposures a day. Refer to the instructions at the bottom of the sheet, explaining that the child placed a checkmark in each circle after completing each exposure. Also, during and/or after exposures, those nasty anxiety symptoms are often present. Discuss with the child that *this is where Jaden and YOU will use your coping techniques that you have in your toolbox*. Point to the instruction, "Color in the circle if you used your coping techniques!" Explain to the child that *the colored circles represent when the Jaden used his techniques. As you get closer to your goal (in this case, handwashing for one minute), OCB isn't bothering you anymore. You will not need to use your coping techniques as you have beat OCB!* You may want to let the child know that for the first few exposures at the desired level, they may still need to use their coping techniques, but eventually, they should not need to.

The final piece is filling out the rewards. This is the fun part! Talk to the child about choosing small daily rewards from their worksheet; Jaden also had a weekly reward which involved completing exposures for six out of seven days, which could be exchanged for going to see a movie!

In addition to the handwashing example, become familiar with two other example **Stepping It Up: Completing My Exposures** sheets on reassurance seeking and gradually moving stuffed animals (Appendices A and B, respectively) to help plan for OCB #1 and subsequent OCBs. For reassurance seeking, note that only two of the three circles were used (one representing morning, one representing evening). In our experience training therapists, having as many exemplars as possible to assist in filling out the various components is helpful.

Explain to the child that it is now time to complete their own homework sheet called **Stepping It Up and Completing My Exposures**. Discuss that they will become very familiar with this worksheet as they begin to boss back several OCBs. These worksheets will help them stay on track and can be used to update and share how things went each week.

Let's break it down into steps:

1. Turn to the blank **Stepping It Up and Completing My Exposures** workbook sheet. Explain all the components (e.g., writing out goals, steps, coping techniques, etc.). Have the child write out the goal or use their preferred modality (e.g., caregiver scribing response).
2. Determine the behavior dimension that will be altered during exposures: duration, frequency, or changing the topography of the OCB (e.g., cutting out pieces of a routine). We suggest preparing for this piece using the **Cognitive Behavioral Skills Template** (Session 2, Appendix A). For examples to support planning exposures, refer to Table 1.1 in Chapter 1, and the example **Stepping It Up and Completing My Exposures** worksheets (Children's Workbook, and Appendix A and B). Designing exposures can be tricky, so reviewing as many examples as you can may be helpful! For the first few OCBs, you will likely write out the daily exposures with input from the child and caregiver. Days written will depend on how your sessions are timed for your clients.
3. Next, list coping techniques. Have the child go back in the workbook and review what they wrote down for all components of Cognitive

Behavior Skills Training. You could ask, *"What are some coping tools or techniques that we just talked about that you think you could use and would help you in fighting OCB?"* It is important that they refer back to the techniques they just listed so their most preferred ones can be included on this sheet. It is quite common for children to talk about bossing back statements, but you may also want to gently remind them of the personalized self-talk for the first OCB based on the exercise **Thinking Differently About OCB** (if appropriate) or additional tools (e.g., deep breathing) that they seemed to like. For the first few OCBs, you will likely take the lead on this piece.

4. You will have reviewed the functional behavior assessment and intervention in Caregiver Module 3 and explored potential replacement behaviors with the child during the **Other Things I Need or Like** activity in the workbook. You may want to refer to this when finalizing coping techniques (e.g., suggestion of talking about a preferred topic with a caregiver if social attention is a function). Encourage the caregiver to talk about the function-based strategies previously discussed and include them in possible coping techniques. As you take the lead, encourage input from the child and caregiver. The more children can talk about these techniques and use them, the more fluent and knowledgeable they will become in what works for them when they are needed.

5. Next, discuss how to check off when exposures are completed. Ensure that you make the connection between doing the coping techniques during and/or after exposures. Refer to **Stepping It Up and Completing My Exposures** examples for variations in recording exposures (e.g., for reassurance seeking, two circles were used for morning and nightly bouts of reassurance). Review instructions with the child and caregiver related to checking circles as well as coloring them in when using coping techniques during and/or after exposures. When the target OCB first reaches the desired levels, coping techniques may still be needed. Eventually, they should not be required by the child. Remind caregivers to encourage children to practice coping techniques when appropriate so they become fluent and can be used for future OCBs.

6. The final piece is choosing rewards. Have the child refer back to their **Rewarding Yourself** and **Small and Big Rewards** workbook sheets to choose daily rewards. It is also optional to have a weekly reward.

7. Maintenance and criteria for moving on to new OCBs is discussed in Session 4. Several pieces of data (e.g., stimulus map, homework and caregiver weekly data can assist with this decision). Keep completing

Stepping It Up and Completing My Exposures sheets (if feasible) for a week at desired levels, with no coping strategies required. If this is not feasible, use other data such as the caregiver's weekly data to determine if further work is needed on previously assigned OCBs.

Token Exchange and Goodbyes

Complete the token exchange where tokens are exchanged for a backup reinforcer from the grab bag. Encourage children to say goodbye to one another (if run in a group format) and/or goodbyes to participating members. Just like in previous sessions, this may need to be modeled and prompted for the first few sessions.

Caregiver Module 3: Introduction to Functional Behavior Assessment and Intervention

Review and Introduction

Distribute new **Caregiver Weekly Data Forms** (Chapter 2, Appendix E). Let caregivers know to bring forward issues or challenges when tackling OCBs, or any new OCBs that arise.

Tell the caregiver that this session's module will focus on the functions of behavior and reviewing their child's completed FBAI.

Instructions

Describe each of the four functions to the caregivers and provide concrete examples:

- Automatic: Internal sensory experience, such as a physical sensation or emotion.
  - Example: A child may engage in handwashing because they enjoy the soothing sensation of the water on their skin and/or because it alleviates anxiety caused by contamination-related obsessions.
- Demand: Avoiding or getting away from an unpreferred or unpleasant demand.
  - Example: A child may engage in ordering their stuffed animals to avoid having to clean up their room when a caregiver has asked them to do it.

- Attention: Accessing attention from or interactions with others.

  - Example: A child may engage in repetitive questioning to seek assurance and access attention from a caregiver.

- Tangible: Accessing a specific tangible item or activity.

  - Example: A child may want to sit in a specific seat because it gives them access to electronic devices.

Explain that children may engage in behaviors to access preferred items (e.g., sensory toys) and/or escape (e.g., an anxiety-inducing situation or task demand). Children can also access these consequences on their own (e.g., arranging their toys in a preferred order) or with the help of someone else (e.g., asking a caregiver to help them turn on the television).

Explain that identifying the function(s) of OCBs beyond escape from anxiety is important for understanding why OCBs happen (e.g., what purpose they serve for that child) and how we can intervene to reduce or eliminate the OCB (e.g., teaching an alternative behavior that may serve the same purpose for the child but is safer and/or more appropriate). These interventions are called function-based interventions.

Next, give each caregiver a copy of their child's completed **Functional Behavior Assessment and Intervention (FBAI) Summary Form** (Session 2, Appendix C). Explain each section of the chart to the caregivers (e.g., compulsions and obsessions, if present; likely functions; function-based interventions) and briefly describe how you arrived at these results.

Helpful hint: A sample of a completed **Functional Behavior Assessment and Intervention Summary Form** has been provided in Session 2 (Appendix D). Refer to this form when modeling and rehearsing the interventions below.

Modeling

Show caregivers how to perform their children's function-based interventions. Have the caregiver or a therapist act as the child as you demonstrate what the intervention will look like.

Two examples of what these demonstrations could look like have been provided in what follows. In your demonstration, it is likely best to replace these templated examples with the child's own OCBs and function-based interventions.

Example 1 (Repetitive Handwashing): Demonstrate what minimizing attention looks like when the child is asking for reassurance. Instead of answering when he asks, "Are my hands clean now?", provide lots of praise when the child does not ask these questions when they usually would. For example, when the child comes in from outside with dirty hands, the caregiver could say "Hey, I love that you came right to the living room rather than washing your hands!" or engage in conversation with them around their special interests (based on preference assessment results, see Session 1), which is a more meaningful way of getting the caregiver's attention.

Example 2 (Arranging Stuffed Animals): Demonstrate what providing alternative access to sensory stimulation looks like. Instead of allowing the child to arrange her stuffed animals, provide her with access to a bin of a select number of sensory toys that she can arrange throughout the day instead. The caregiver can help her use bossing-back statements, like "I can do this!", or model "counting down" coping exercises if needed. When she does start arranging the sensory toys instead of her stuffed animals, provide lots of praise or access to a reinforcer based on the completed preference assessment (see Session 1).

Rehearsal

Provide caregivers with the opportunity to practice taking the lead on the intervention. In group therapy, this can be done one at a time or by dividing caregivers into pairs (e.g., one caregiver pretends to be the child while the other implements the intervention, and then the roles are reversed).

If rehearsal isn't possible, tell the caregiver that this can be reviewed thoroughly during individual programming for OCBs later in the session.

All functions of OCBs are important to address; however, addressing socially mediated functions through function-based strategies is the primary focus of Caregiver Module 3. Escape from anxiety functions will be addressed in greater detail in Caregiver Module 5.

Feedback

Provide positive and specific praise when the caregiver demonstrates the intervention correctly (e.g., "You've implemented that strategy perfectly!") and corrective feedback for incorrect/incomplete components (e.g., "Remember to ensure you give praise immediately after the replacement behavior").

Scheduling Follow-Up Meetings

Review the FBAI worksheet for the new OCB. If needed, continue to review the completed FBAI for the OCB during individualized programming. Take a few minutes to schedule follow-up meetings with caregivers to complete the functional behavior assessments for the next OCB (see Chapter 3 for details). Finalize which OCB will be the focus of the upcoming session.

Additional Therapist Preparation for Session 4

- Review Sample **Stepping It Up and Completing My Exposures** sheets.
- Complete planning using the **Cognitive Behavioral Skills Template** (Session 2, Appendix A).
- Complete the **Functional Behavior Assessment and Intervention (FBAI) Summary Form** (Session 2, Appendix C) for the next OCB to be targeted (add to the existing FBAI Summary Form).

Sample Stepping It Up Worksheet: Asking for Reassurance

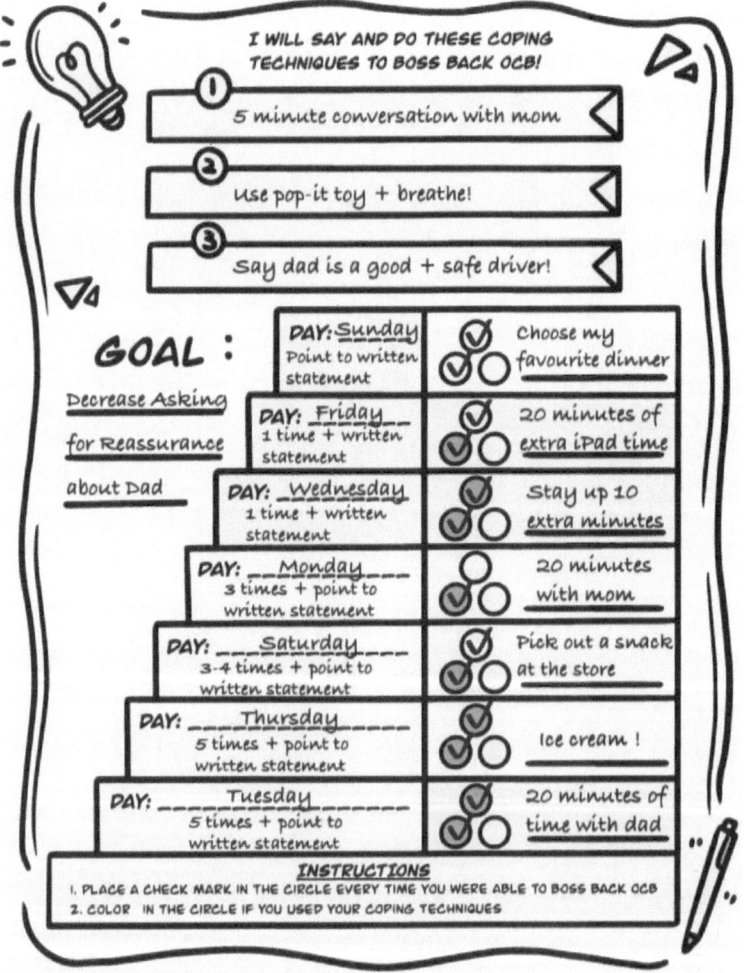

Appendix B

Sample Stepping It Up Worksheet: Ordering Stuffed Animals

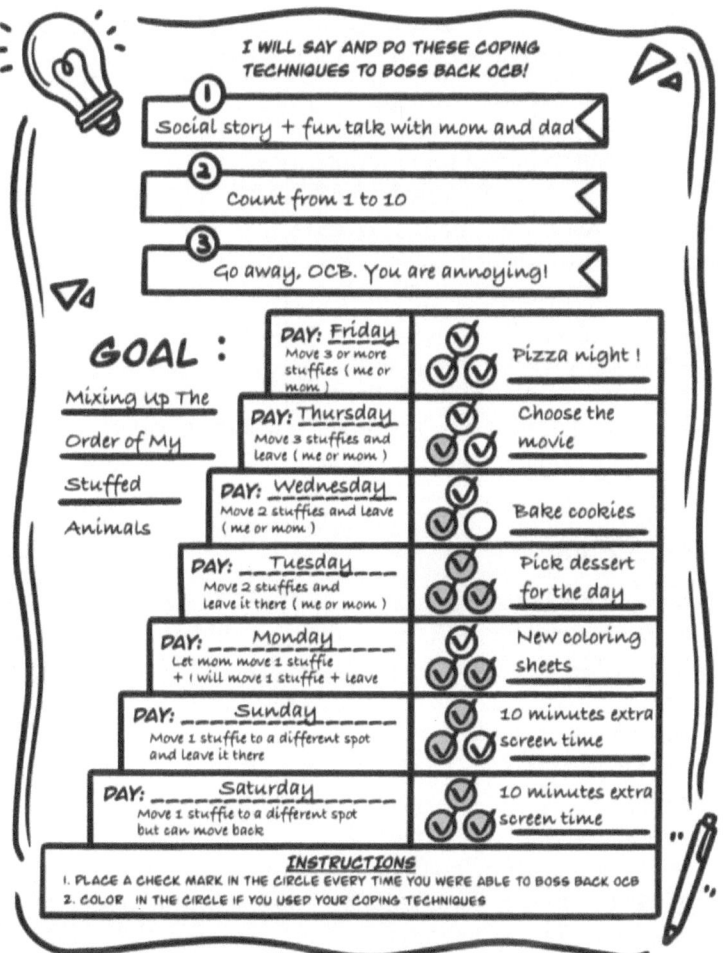

I WILL SAY AND DO THESE COPING TECHNIQUES TO BOSS BACK OCB!

1. Social story + fun talk with mom and dad
2. Count from 1 to 10
3. Go away, OCB. You are annoying!

GOAL: Mixing Up The Order of My Stuffed Animals

DAY: Friday
Move 3 or more stuffies (me or mom)
Pizza night !

DAY: Thursday
Move 3 stuffies and leave (me or mom)
Choose the movie

DAY: Wednesday
Move 2 stuffies and leave (me or mom)
Bake cookies

DAY: Tuesday
Move 2 stuffies and leave it there (me or mom)
Pick dessert for the day

DAY: Monday
Let mom move 1 stuffie + I will move 1 stuffie + leave
New coloring sheets

DAY: Sunday
Move 1 stuffie to a different spot and leave it there
10 minutes extra screen time

DAY: Saturday
Move 1 stuffie to a different spot but can move back
10 minutes extra screen time

INSTRUCTIONS
1. PLACE A CHECK MARK IN THE CIRCLE EVERY TIME YOU WERE ABLE TO BOSS BACK OCB
2. COLOR IN THE CIRCLE IF YOU USED YOUR COPING TECHNIQUES

Chapter 9

Session 4

Progress Review of First OCB and Tackling New OCBs

Materials

- Children's Workbook
- Flipchart/Whiteboard
- Token Board (Session 1, Appendix A)
- Tokens and grab bag of preferred items
- Activities/food items for break/snack
- ABC Narrative Form (Chapter 3, Appendix B)
- Reinforcer Checklist (Chapter 1, Appendix B)
- Cognitive Behavioral Skills Template (Session 2, Appendix A)
- Drawing and Sharing a Seasonal Picture materials (e.g., crayons, markers, felt, construction paper)
- Blank Caregiver Weekly Data Form (Chapter 2, Appendix E)
- Obsession and Compulsion Recording Template (Chapter 2, Appendix B)
- Operational Definitions and Interference Handout (Chapter 2, Appendix C)

Session Outline

- Homework Review (20 Min.)
- Social Skills Activity: Alphabet Game (15 Min.)
- Review of Previous Work on the First OCB and Further Programming (20 Min.)
- Break and Snack (10 Min.)
- Social Skills Activity: Drawing and Sharing a Seasonal Picture (15 Min.)
- Individualized Intervention for OCB #2 and Homework (35 Min.)
- Token Exchange and Goodbyes (5 Min.)
- Caregiver Module 4: Functional Behavior Assessment and FBAI: Special Topic on Setting Events (25 Min.) – To take place during Break and Snack, and Drawing and Sharing a Seasonal Picture

DOI: 10.4324/9781003410126-9

Pre-Session Checklist

- Arrange the environment (e.g., seating) as you feel appropriate.
- You may continue to outline the session activities on a whiteboard or flipchart.
- Have child **Token Boards** ready with prosocial behaviors written on them. Vary tokens to depict preferred pictures or stickers to maintain interest.
- Complete the **Cognitive Behavioral Skills Template** (Session 2, Appendix A) for next target OCB.
- Prepare new **Caregiver Weekly Data Forms** (Chapter 2, Appendix E).
- Complete the **Functional Behavior Assessment and Intervention (FBAI) Summary Form** (based on functional behavior assessment completed) for next target OCB (Session 2, Appendix C).

Session Implementation

Homework Review

Review today's schedule and hand out the **Token Boards** (Session 1, Appendix A) with prosocial behaviors written on them for today's session. Use the first few minutes to collect **Caregiver Weekly Data Forms** (Chapter 2, Appendix E) from the previous week. Have children give a brief report of progress on their first obsessive-compulsive behavior (OCB). Ask caregivers to participate as appropriate. Leading prompts may be provided to the children, such as *"Talk about something that you are proud of"* or *"Name something that went well this week."* Alternatively, you could ask children to comment on how their exposures went or whether they accessed the rewards they wrote down. If not volunteered, you may ask what coping techniques they used and if they were helpful. As you progress through sessions, caregiver and therapist prompts and support may be faded so that children become increasingly independent in vocalizing their experiences. Ideally, this discussion becomes more open-ended as children become more comfortable and confident in sharing material.

Ask children to turn to the **Mapping OCB** sheet from Session 2. Using the stimulus map, the **Caregiver Weekly Data Forms** (Chapter 2, Appendix E), and the completed **Stepping It Up: Completing My Exposures** sheet, discuss progress and obstacles with the targeted OCB. These will also provide insight into whether a new target OCB should be added. Further, this time can be used to discuss a possible target OCB for Session 5 and whether a functional behavior assessment should be completed for the next session. This should be discussed further with caregivers in Caregiver Module 4.

Ask the child, *Should [Targeted OCB] be moved on the stimulus map or does it need to be worked on a little bit more?* Assist the child or youth in making this decision and emphasize that with a lot of kids, it takes a bit of time before behaviors move to the right on the map and you outsmart OCB! See definitions of stimulus map zones in Session 2 if you need a brief review. You may also refer to our suggestions for definitions of minimal and good progress in helping the child decide whether the compulsion moves over on the stimulus map to be closer to the Me Zone (see Session 2). Some OCBs may move back and forth between zones if re-emergence occurs.

Box 9.1   Reminder!

Remember to give behavior-specific praise and deliver tokens as appropriate throughout the session.

Suggested Criteria for Moving to the Next OCB

Use the data (**Caregiver Weekly Data Forms**, stimulus map, **Stepping It Up: Completing My Exposures** sheets) and a discussion with the caregiver and child to decide whether to program for a second OCB in this session. Over one week, if progress is being made, you should see some movement toward desired levels on the caregiver rating sheet for individual OCBs (e.g., a rating of five to a rating of three over several days). Also, the child should show increased fluency in using the coping techniques and indicate some success in resisting the OCB (which would be indicated by several successful attempts on Exposure/Response Prevention (E/RP) steps and using coping techniques). The stimulus map can be used for discussion and assessing progress.

1. Minimal Progress: If the criteria are not met, the team (child, caregiver, therapist) may make the joint decision to continue working on the same OCB for the following week. If the child is very motivated but has made minimal progress, you may continue working on OCB #1 and introduce a new OCB. As indicated in Chapter 1, we found that children remained focused and were not overwhelmed if we were actively working on no more than two OCBs at a time.
2. Good Progress: If the child has made good progress with the first OCB and the urge to complete it is gone (as evidenced by it being at desired levels for most days with no need to use coping techniques), you may discontinue data collection (i.e., filling out a **Stepping It Up:**

Completing My Exposures worksheet). However, it is more likely that the child may have made some progress, but you encourage continued work on OCB #1. For example, in the **Stepping It Up: Completing My Exposures** for Jaden's handwashing (Workbook, Session 3), the child reduced handwashing to one minute (desired level) with no need for coping techniques, but only for the last day. It is helpful to continue collecting data for one extra week to ensure the urge to do the compulsion is gone. Review and modify the intervention (if necessary) and then complete another **Stepping It Up: Completing My Exposures** worksheet (see below for step-by-step details).

Encourage generalization to other stimuli, settings, and people as appropriate. For example, in the case of handwashing, have the child use different sinks in the home setting. However, if there is anxiety or distress associated with other stimuli, settings, and people, an individual program plan may be needed.

After the break and Caregiver Module, you will develop a new individualized treatment plan for OCB #2 on a second **Stepping It Up: Completing My Exposures** sheet. If not moving on, more time can be spent problem-solving OCB #1 and reviewing coping techniques for OCB #1 and future OCBs.

Social Skills Activity: Alphabet Game

The Alphabet Game requires children to move their bodies to mimic different letters of the alphabet. This is an intermediate social skill activity (see Chapter 4 for further details).

Instructions: Have the children stand in a circle. Inform the children that they will be making shapes using their bodies. Model the activity first by choosing a letter and using your body to make that shape. Encourage the children to copy you. Next, go around the circle so that each child has a turn to choose a letter and demonstrate the shape. Children can use the first letter of their name or choose their favorite letter. Encourage the children to copy each child as they demonstrate the shape. Continue until each child has had a turn.

In a one-on-one setting, the therapist or caregivers can participate in the activity by making the letters of the alphabet alongside the child. See Chapter 4 for additional modifications.

Review of Previous Work on the First OCB and Further Programming

Take this time to review the previous work on OCBs and continue programming as needed. We have found it helpful to build off the discussion at the beginning of the session on OCB #1 to provide a connection with the previous material discussed. If applicable, bring up something the child or caregiver noted that they were proud of regarding the child's work on the OCB.

Here are some suggested steps for reviewing programming:

- Turn to the completed E/RP worksheet and flip to the blank E/RP sheet in the Children's Workbook. Have your **Cognitive Behavioral Skills Template** (Session 2, Appendix A) prepared.

- Review the goal, behavior dimension, and E/RP steps that were part of the gradual exposure. Reflect on the steps written on the **Stepping It Up: Completing My Exposures** sheet for OCB #1. Begin by examining whether steps need to be adjusted in any way (e.g., do steps need to be added at certain points or is the child ready to move onto a more challenging step?). You can gauge this by looking at the progress (checkmarks) for exposures and colored circles indicating the children engaged in their replacement behaviors. If very little is filled in, this may also be a discussion to have. This can include exploring child motivation, time to complete exposures that week, and other variables relevant to the child and their family (e.g., stresses, family dynamics). Modify as needed to make it feasible for the child and caregivers.

  - Example: In the example **Stepping It Up: Completing My Exposures** case of handwashing (Session 3), the child is making good progress and is down to one minute (desired level). The new **Stepping It Up: Completing My Exposures** sheet could include all steps at one minute and fading out coping techniques given the lessened urge to engage in the OCB. Have the child assist in filling in their steps and days of the week. Alternatively, the child may have made minimal progress and is stuck at washing for five minutes instead of the initial ten minutes. In this case, you may consider making the steps smaller (reducing the increments between each step or making the reinforcer larger to aid motivation to complete exposures). You may also look at setting events (see Caregiver Module 4 and Chapter 3). Was the child ill that week or did they have a challenging week at school? Depending on the setting events, you may modify the plan accordingly to ensure success. You may convey to the caregiver that if the child does not feel successful or there are no fun things embedded in the program, they may not continue with treatment.

- Using the completed **Stepping It Up: Completing My Exposures** sheet, have the child review the coping techniques they wrote down. If helpful, turn to the coping techniques written down in Session 3 for OCB #1 and review the types of coping techniques checked off or preferred by the child. Here are the four types of coping techniques:

- *Believing in Myself: What I Can Do and Say to OCB*
- *My Toolbox*
- *Other Things I Need or Like*
- *Thinking Differently and Outsmarting OCB*

- Note that the **Functional Behavior Assessment and Intervention (FBAI) Summary Form** (which supports the **Other Things I Need or Like** activity) will be reviewed in the Caregiver Module.
- Use the completed **Stepping It Up: Completing My Exposures** sheet and Session 3 worksheets on coping techniques for OCB #1 to talk about what worked from the child and caregiver's views. Can existing components be expanded upon? Are there other coping techniques that could be used? Have the child fill in their coping techniques on the new **Stepping It Up: Completing My Exposures** sheet for what they will do and say to boss back OCB this week.
- Emphasize the connection between completing coping techniques during and/or after completing exposure and response prevention steps (and coloring in the circles). This will be worked on in Caregiver Module 5 to support current and future OCBs. In our experience, knowing when and how to be flexible with the use of coping techniques is sometimes a challenge for caregivers and children.
- Last, fill out the rewards by referring to the completed **Rewarding Yourself** and **Small and Big Rewards** worksheets or choosing from the options on the completed **Stepping It Up: Completing My Exposures** sheet from last week. Explore what the children liked and if they received the reward the same day as completing the exposure. Brainstorm preferred items to add based on their current interests. If OCB programming is at desired levels (and you are making sure this remains for approximately a week), you may want to encourage the child to choose smaller reinforcers and remind them that they will be picking rewards for OCB #2, as well. Keep in mind while planning intervention that you want to ensure that you save the powerful ones for the bigger challenges!

Therapist Reflection on Challenges

- Overall, we suggest that you examine whether challenges are related to incorrect or little use of strategies or other variables. If challenges are related to the incorrect use of strategies, model and practice as appropriate. If challenges are related to limited use of strategies, does response effort need to be reduced or the program intensity adjusted?

- Attend to whether new thoughts surrounding the compulsion have been identified. You could also probe for additional thoughts as part of reviewing the **Thinking Differently and Outsmarting OCB** activity. Additional work in the cognitive restructuring area may be beneficial.
- Note setting events and antecedents that children and youth discuss as this will aid in obtaining a better understanding of the OCB and progress made. Pay attention to variables such as noise levels, task materials, time of day, verbal demands, the absence of attention, and illness, to name a few.

Note: At this point, children will complete Break and Snack (10 Min.) and Social Skills Activity: Drawing and Sharing a Seasonal Picture (15 Min.) while Caregivers complete Caregiver Module 4: Functional Behavior Assessment and FBAI: Special Topic on Setting Events (25 Min.)

Break and Snack

You may continue to offer snacks from the **Reinforcer Checklist** (Chapter 1, Appendix B). Depending on your policies, snacks may be prepared ahead of time or caregivers may be asked to bring in snacks.

Allow this break period to be child-directed (e.g., a child may want to draw or attempt to initiate a game with you). You can capitalize on this time to build rapport with the children or facilitate rapport building within the group. If helpful, use a timer and give children reminders of the time remaining.

You may use this time to observe OCBs or contrive situations to collect descriptive data (if possible) using the **ABC Narrative Form** (Chapter 3, Appendix B) or you may use one of your own.

Social Skills Activity: Drawing and Sharing a Seasonal Picture

Drawing and sharing seasonal pictures involves children using various art mediums (e.g., crayons, markers, felt, construction paper) to create a seasonal picture. This is an intermediate social skill activity (see Chapter 4 for further details).

Instructions: Ask the children to think of what they like about this time of year (e.g., smelling flowers, going to the beach, jumping in leaf piles, building snowmen, depending on the season!). If group therapy, divide the children into small groups and provide each group with a set of art supplies to share (e.g., markers, stickers, stencils). Ask the children to use their imaginations to create a seasonal picture. Once everyone is finished, encourage each child to share their picture with their group. If a child is hesitant, they may show their picture to a therapist or another child. After each child has shown their picture, encourage the group to compliment them and share what they liked about their picture.

In a one-on-one setting, the child may informally share and discuss their picture with the therapist and/or caregivers. See Chapter 4 for additional modifications.

Individualized Intervention for OCB #2 and Homework

If not moving on to OCB #2, review OCB #1 as needed.

Refer to your completed **Cognitive Behavioral Skills Template** (Session 2, Appendix A) for OCB #2. Have children complete the **OCB News** for the second OCB. Given the different types of coping techniques are still new to most children and it is a new OCB to address, it is suggested that you go through each worksheet in the workbook for Session 4 with the new OCB. In our experience, exposure often aided in children choosing new techniques. They also became more creative and confident in choosing their coping techniques! For Session 4, continue structured programming and provide as much assistance as needed. Likely, you will still be guiding the child and caregiver through these activities. There will be plenty of time for fading your guidance as sessions progress.

Believing in Myself: What I Can Do and Say to OCB

In Sessions 1 to 3, children were taught to tell OCB to go away; for example, "Beat it!" or simply acknowledge OCB's presence (e.g., "Hi there, OCB" [nickname]). You are teaching the child to either boss back OCB or to accept OCB's presence and be OK with it. For the second OCB, you will begin with the activity **Believing in Myself: What I Can Do and Say to OCB** in the workbook. Have children continue to write out or draw bossing-back statements on the lines or in the thought bubbles. Talk about OCB #2 with reference to the recently completed **OCB News** and discuss the compulsion and thought (if possible). Encourage the child to say the statements out loud (if comfortable) and picture themselves bossing back OCB. Some children get very creative with role-playing and different statements at this stage. Other children like to write down or draw similar statements to the first OCB.

Note that they can also write things they can "do" to OCB such as "I'm going to beat you up, OCB!" or "Here's a karate move for you!" if they are focusing more on what they can say. Have the children build on or generate a few new responses and then move on to the next technique.

My Toolbox

Review the **My Toolbox** activity and the coping strategies (with pictures). There are likely plenty that have not been explored. Some may be more applicable for some OCBs than others; you may have brainstormed this with your **Cognitive Behavioral Skills Template** and can offer suggestions, or the child may have ideas related to OCB #2. Please note that there are also blank squares for children to generate their own.

You may ask, *What worked for the last OCB? What did you not try?* Does the child and their support team think that any new techniques listed would fit well as replacement behaviors? Choose one or two techniques to focus on for the second OCB. Similar to Session 3, have them practice the technique and place a checkmark in the box after attempting it. Model the technique and provide prompting as needed. Encourage the caregiver to discuss and model the technique or provide prompting at home with praise for the child.

Other Things I Need or Like

Referring to the **Functional Behavior Assessment and Intervention (FBAI) Summary Form,** complete the **Other Things I Need or Like** activity. Connect FBAI strategies to visuals in the workbook (e.g., having a conversation if social attention was a function; playing with things that look and feel good if the compulsion provided automatic sensory stimulation). Given the caregiver has now participated in a few caregiver modules exploring functions of behavior, try to have them take a more extensive lead in this piece and provide prompts as needed. For example, in Session 3 we discussed social attention as a function and engaging in conversation rather than the compulsion (e.g., asking for reassurance and the caregiver providing it). This could be planned out by the caregiver (e.g., topics, engaging in conversation while the child is anxious during the compulsion or after completing their exposure step). This is just one example of many. These strategies can be written in the child's workbook, or notes could be made on the **Functional Behavior Assessment and Intervention (FBAI) Summary Form**. Caregivers have reported that returning to these materials post-treatment can help maintain a positive treatment response.

Thinking Differently and Self-Talk to Outsmart OCB

The **Thinking Differently and Outsmarting My OCB** activity is the final set of cognitive and behavioral skills. You need to use your discretion as to how much time you spend on this activity. See Chapter 1, Thinking Differently: Cognitive Restructuring for a more detailed description of cognitive restructuring and self-talk. Many school-age children have a difficult time articulating the obsessions or thoughts and physiological sensations that precede compulsions. You may attempt to restructure or reframe thoughts if appropriate and the child's cognitive and developmental profile allows for it. Depending on the OCB, you may be able to do some cognitive restructuring and reframing of thoughts. Children can become more aware of and comfortable talking about thoughts as treatment progresses. This should be individualized for each child. Session 3 offers additional examples that may be suitable for the child you are working with and the OCB.

For children who do not have a thought or perhaps have a partial thought that would be difficult to work with, you may move to the part of the worksheet on **Outsmarting my OCB.** As mentioned in Session 3, we differentiate these self-talk statements from externalizing statements as they are statements or rules specific to the targeted OCB. They may build off knowledge learned in cognitive restructuring, or they may be rules that the child follows that are specific to the OCB (e.g., "I can leave my snow gear at home because it's summertime and it will make me sweat"). Last, you may spend time replacing negative self-statements with positive self-statements. The example we gave in Session 3 was a child saying, "I have to check the door five times. I can't stop." The "I can't" may be a theme for many OCBs. You may try to replace this with "I can do it. I'm not going to let OCB beat me" OR "I'm just going to check three times. I'm on my way to outsmarting OCB!" Perhaps in this session, you can have the child be more involved in creating their own personalized OCB statements!

Rewarding Yourself

Have the child turn to the **Rewarding Yourself** activities in the workbook. Read the text aloud or have the child or caregiver do so. Explain that "saying no to OCB" or resisting the urge to do a compulsion can be hard. Say something like, *it's time to write down some rewards you can work for when completing your exposures, and say no to OCB!* Explain to children that they will write daily rewards on their homework sheet to earn when they're being brave and bossing back OCB. Try to make the connection for them between the rewards and completing their exposures (and using their coping techniques) each day.

If they need assistance, have their **Reinforcer Checklist** (see Chapter 1, Appendix B) available. Preferences do change frequently for some children and youth, so it can be helpful to readminister it. In our experience, children are often good at generating tangible rewards based on things they engage in daily (e.g., iPad use). Some other examples include spending 15–20 min doing their activity of choice with a caregiver or choosing their favorite meal for dinner. The child does not need to fill out all five rewards. Come up with a few and then move on to the next page. Immediate reinforcement is better than delayed reinforcement. Therefore, children will choose daily rewards for completing exposures. Explain to the caregiver and child that many of the rewards should be small rewards that can be delivered each day. See Chapter 1, Adaptations Embedded into Functional Behavior-based Cognitive Behavioral Therapy (Fb-CBT) for more information on reinforcement.

Small and Big Rewards

Sometimes children have a difficult time separating small rewards from big rewards. The **Small and Big Rewards** can be used to explore different types of rewards that can be differentially delivered daily versus at the end of the week, or for easier homework tasks compared to more challenging tasks. Big rewards can be given at the end of the week contingent on the child's success throughout the week (and the delivery of daily rewards). Given the focus on small rewards on the **Rewarding Yourself** sheet, you may want to encourage children to copy what they have already generated. If you have generated sufficient information in the **Rewarding Yourself** activity, you may choose to skip this sheet. You can refer to this sheet when completing the **Stepping It Up: Completing My Exposures** homework to identify small rewards for daily practice and large rewards for sustained success.

Completing E/RP Worksheet for OCB #2

Explain to the child that it is now time to complete their homework sheet called **Stepping It Up and Completing My Exposures**. They will become familiar with this routine as the sessions progress. These worksheets will help them stay on track, look at their progress, and share their wins!

1. Turn to the blank **Stepping It Up and Completing My Exposures** workbook sheet. Explain all the components (e.g., writing out goals, steps, coping techniques, etc.). Have the child write out the goal or use their preferred modality (e.g., caregiver scribing response).
2. Determine the behavior dimension that will be altered during exposures: duration, frequency, or changing the topography of the OCB (e.g., cutting out pieces of a routine). We suggest preparing for this piece using the **Cognitive Behavioral Skills Template** (Session 2, Appendix A). For examples to support planning exposures, refer to Table 1.1 in Chapter 1, and the example **Stepping It Up and Completing My Exposures** worksheets (Children's Workbook, and Appendix A and B, Chapter 3). Write out the daily exposures with input from the child and caregiver.

3. List coping techniques. Have the child go back in the workbook and review what they wrote down for all components of Cognitive Behavior Skills Training. You could ask, *"What are some coping tools or techniques that we just talked about that you think you could use and would help you in fighting OCB?"* It is important that they refer back to the techniques they just listed so their most preferred ones can be included on this sheet. You can build off the discussion you just had for OCB #1. They may also want to try new techniques.

4. You will have reviewed the functional behavior assessment and intervention in Caregiver Module 4 and explored potential replacement behaviors with the child during the **Other Things I Need or Like** activity in the workbook. You may want to refer to this when finalizing coping techniques (e.g., suggestion of talking about a preferred topic with a caregiver if social attention is a function).

5. Next, discuss how to check off when exposure steps are completed. Tell children and caregivers that coping techniques should be used during and/or after exposures. Review instructions with the child and caregiver related to checking circles as well as coloring them in when using coping techniques during and/or after exposures. When the target OCB first reaches the desired levels, coping techniques may still be needed. Eventually, they should not be required by the child. Remind caregivers to encourage children to practice coping techniques when appropriate so they become fluent and can be used for future OCBs.

6. The final step is choosing rewards. Have the child refer back to their **Rewarding Yourself** and **Small and Big Rewards** workbook sheets to choose daily rewards. It is also optional to have a weekly reward.

Maintenance and criteria for moving on to new OCBs are discussed at the beginning of this session. Several pieces of data (e.g., stimulus map, **Stepping It Up and Completing My Exposures** homework, and **Caregiver Weekly Data Forms**) can assist with this decision. Keep completing **Stepping It Up and Completing My Exposures** sheets (if feasible) for a week at desired levels, with no coping strategies required. If this is not feasible, use other data such as the caregiver's weekly data to determine if further work is needed on previously assigned OCBs.

Token Exchange and Goodbyes

Complete the token exchange and have the children say goodbye to one another.

Caregiver Module 4: Functional Behavior Assessment and FBAI: Special Topic on Setting Events

Review and Introduction

Distribute new **Caregiver Weekly Data Forms** (Chapter 2, Appendix E). Let caregivers know to bring forward issues or challenges when tackling OCBs, or any new OCBs that arise.

Tell the caregivers that this week's module will focus on reviewing their child's completed FBAI and function-based strategies.

Instruction

Provide each caregiver with an updated copy of their child's completed **Functional Behavior Assessment and Intervention (FBAI) Summary Form** (Session 2, Appendix C).

First, ask caregivers if they have any questions or if they would like to review any of the function-based interventions taught last week. If they do, focus on providing guidance before moving on to the next section.

Next, describe setting events and provide concrete examples:

- Setting events are circumstances that lead to an increased likelihood of OCBs occurring.
- Circumstances that may act as setting events for a child: Lack of sleep, illness, disruptions in routine, overstimulation, or feelings of deprivation (e.g., the child is deprived of attention because they haven't seen the caregiver all day).

Setting events can be internal (e.g., the child is ill) or external (e.g., the child experiences a disruption in their routine). They can happen immediately before the OCB (e.g., a child who has the predisposition for rearranging acquires a new stuffed animal) or far in advance (e.g., a child with contamination-related compulsions has been sick for the past week).

It is important for the caregivers to be aware of setting events that may impact their child's OCBs because it may influence their expectations and when they implement the function-based interventions. For example, if a child is exceptionally muddy (a rare occurrence for this child), you may not want to progress to a more difficult handwashing exposure at that very moment. If a child is sick, you might provide additional assistance to help the child reduce arranging that day.

Modeling

Show caregivers how to modify their child's function-based interventions when a setting event is present. Have the caregiver or a therapist act as the child as you demonstrate what the modification will look like.

Two examples of what these demonstrations could look like are provided. In your demonstration, it is likely best to replace these templated examples with the child's OCBs, setting events, and function-based interventions.

Example 1 (Repetitive Handwashing): Demonstrate how to move back a step during handwashing exposures (in other words, decrease the expectation) when the child is exceptionally muddy. For instance, offer the child the choice of staying at the current step (handwashing for four minutes) or returning to a previously mastered step (e.g., six minutes). If the child chooses to challenge themself by staying at the current step and is successful, provide more attention than usual, multiple reinforcers, and/or longer access to a reinforcer based on the completed preference assessment (see Chapter 1).

Example 2 (Arranging Stuffed Animals): Demonstrate how to provide additional assistance (e.g., increasing prompts) to a sick child who is working on reducing arranging and ordering of stuffed animals. For instance, if the child has a sore stomach, their tolerance for moving through gradual exposure steps may be lower than usual. During the exposure (e.g., moving the stuffed animal out of order and then back into place), you may provide more assistance while the stuffed animal is out of order with the coping technique (e.g., counting from one to ten together in a sing-song manner) rather than expecting them to do this independently. If the child is successful, provide lots of praise, multiple reinforcers, and/or longer access to a reinforcer for overcoming their anxiety or distress despite feeling under the weather (see Chapters 1 and 2).

Rehearsal

Provide caregivers with the opportunity to practice taking the lead on the intervention. In group therapy, this can be done one at a time or by dividing caregivers into pairs (e.g., one caregiver pretends to be the child while the other implements the intervention, and then the roles are reversed).

If rehearsal isn't possible, tell the caregiver that this will be reviewed thoroughly during individual programming for OCBs later in the session.

Feedback

Provide positive and specific praise when the caregiver demonstrates the intervention correctly (e.g., "You've modified that intervention perfectly!") and corrective feedback for incorrect/incomplete components (e.g., "You could make that step even easier for [Child's Name]").

Scheduling Follow-Up Meetings

Review the FBAI worksheet for the new OCB. If needed, continue to review the completed FBAI for the OCB during individualized programming. Take a few minutes to schedule follow-up meetings with caregivers to complete the functional behavior assessments for the next OCB (see Chapter 3 for details). Finalize which OCB will be the focus of the upcoming session.

Chapter 10

Session 5

Continued OCB Mapping and Gradually Moving Up the Hierarchy

Materials

- Children's Workbook
- Flipchart/Whiteboard
- Token Board (Session 1, Appendix A)
- Tokens and grab bag of preferred items
- Cognitive Behavioral Skills Template (Session 2, Appendix A)
- Activities/food items for break/snack
- ABC Narrative Form (Chapter 3, Appendix B)
- Reinforcer Checklist (Chapter 1, Appendix B)
- Freestyle Building construction materials (e.g., building blocks, LEGO®) and pictures of different structures the children will build
- Miniature sticky notes or paper and scissors to write and cut out a list of child compulsions
- Blank Caregiver Weekly Data Form (Chapter 2, Appendix E)
- Operational Definitions and Interference Handout (Chapter 2, Appendix C)

Session Outline

- Homework Review (20 Min.)
- Review of Previous Work on OCBs and Further Programming (20 Min.)
- Break and Snack (10 Min.)
- Social Skills Activity: Freestyle Building (15 Min.)
- Examining Quality of Life (15 Min.)
- Individualized Intervention for OCB #3 and Homework (35 Min.)
- Token Exchange and Goodbyes (5 Min.)
- Caregiver Module 5: Functional Behavior Assessment and FBAI: Special Topic on Addressing Dual Functions (25 Min.) – To take place during Break and Snack, and Freestyle Building

DOI: 10.4324/9781003410126-10

Pre-Session Checklist

- Arrange the environment (e.g., seating) as you feel appropriate.
- You may continue to outline the session activities on a whiteboard or flipchart.
- Have child token sheets ready with prosocial behaviors written on them. Vary tokens to depict preferred pictures or stickers to maintain interest.
- Preplanning with Cognitive Behavioral Skills Template for OCBs (see Session 2, Appendix A).
- Have new caregiver data sheets ready (Chapter 2, Appendix E).
- Complete the FBAI Summary Form (based on FBA completed this last week) (Session 2, Appendix C).

Session Implementation

Homework Review

Use the first few minutes to collect **Caregiver Weekly Data Forms** (Chapter 2, Appendix E) from the previous week. Review today's schedule and hand out the **Token Boards** (Session 1, Appendix A) with prosocial behaviors written on them for today's session. Then, have children match the words with the correct answers and answer the questions on the **Homework Review** activity in the workbook. Review and comment as appropriate.

Have children give a brief review of progress with their first two obsessive-compulsive behaviors (OCBs). Ask caregivers to continue to participate as appropriate. Leading prompts may be given to the children, "*Talk about something that you are proud of,*" or "*Name something that went well this week.*" Alternatively, you could ask children to comment on how their exposures went or whether they accessed the rewards they wrote down. If not volunteered, you may ask what coping techniques they used and if they were helpful. Encourage children to become increasingly independent in vocalizing their experiences. Learners will have a range of cognitive, developmental, and socio-emotional skills. In each session, try to ask for a little more detail or have them build on their expressive language. Ask children to turn to the **Mapping OCB** sheet from Session 2. Using the stimulus map, the **Caregiver Weekly Data Forms** (Chapter 2, Appendix E), and the completed **Stepping It Up: Completing My Exposures** sheets, discuss progress and obstacles with the targeted OCBs. Further, this time can be used to discuss possible target OCBs for Session 6 and whether a functional behavior assessment should be completed for the next session. This should be discussed with caregivers further in Caregiver Module 5.

Ask the child, *Should [Targeted OCBs] be moved on the stimulus map or do they need to be worked on a little bit more?* Assist the child or youth in making this decision and emphasize that some OCBs take more time than others and move a bit slower to the Me Zone. See definitions of stimulus map zones in Session 2 if you need a brief review. You may also refer to our definitions of minimal and good progress in helping the child to decide whether the compulsion moves over on the stimulus map to be closer to the Me Zone. Some OCBs may move back and forth between zones if re-emergence occurs.

Now that children are familiar with OCBs and strategies to address them, you can discuss the interference of OCBs and how they can impact the quality of life for themselves and their family members. This may increase motivation to continue to engage in treatment and reinforce the need to learn the coping techniques to tackle OCBs when they arise. The Quality of Life exercise later in the session explores this further.

Box 10.1   Reminder!

Remember to give behavior-specific praise and deliver tokens as appropriate throughout the session.

Suggested Criteria for Moving to the Next OCB

Use the data (**Caregiver Weekly Data Forms**, stimulus map, **Stepping It Up: Completing My Exposures** sheets) and a discussion with the caregiver and child to decide whether to program for an additional OCB in this session. Over one week, if progress is being made, you should see some movement toward desired levels on the caregiver rating sheet for individual OCBs (e.g., a rating of five to a rating of three over several days). Also, the child should show increased fluency in using the coping techniques and indicate some success in resisting the OCB (which would be indicated by several successful attempts on Exposure/ Response Prevention (E/RP) steps and using coping techniques). The stimulus map can be used for discussion and assessing progress.

1. Minimal Progress: If the criteria are not met, the team (child, caregiver, therapist) may make the joint decision to continue working on the same OCBs for the following week. You are now at the point

where you are reviewing progress for two OCBs. If the child has made minimal progress on both OCBs, consider pausing here and continuing to refine intervention plans for both OCBs. In some instances, we have paused intervention for one OCB given a contributing variable (e.g., a family stressor that is preventing child exposures at home) and have continued to work on the other and/or introduced an alternative OCB.

2. Good Progress: If the child has made good progress with the first OCB and the urge to complete it is gone (as evidenced by it being at desired levels for most days with no need to use coping techniques), you may discontinue data collection (i.e., filling out a **Stepping It Up: Completing My Exposures** worksheet). If the child has also made good progress with the second OCB and the urge to complete it is gone (as evidenced by it being at desired levels for most days with no need for coping techniques), you may discontinue data collection. However, one week is usually not enough. It will be more likely that the child made some progress, but you encourage continued work on OCB #2 to ensure the urge is completely gone (see case of handwashing described in Session 3). Review and modify the intervention (if necessary) and then complete another **Stepping It Up: Completing My Exposures** worksheet. See below for step-by-step details.

Encourage generalization to other stimuli, settings, and people as appropriate. For example, in the case of handwashing, have the child use different sinks in the home setting. However, if there is anxiety or distress associated with other stimuli, settings, and people, an individual program plan may be needed.

After the break and Caregiver Module, you will develop a new individualized treatment plan for OCB #3 on a second **Stepping It Up: Completing My Exposures** worksheet. If not moving on, you can discuss the previous OCBs and review coping techniques.

Review of Previous Work on OCBs and Further Programming

Take this time to review the previous work on OCBs and continue programming as needed. By this session, child and youth are often becoming increasingly fluent in choosing and utilizing coping techniques while completing exposure steps.

Here are some suggested steps for reviewing programming:

- Review the completed **Stepping It Up: Completing My Exposures** sheet and begin working on a new **Stepping It Up: Completing My**

Exposures in the workbook. Have your **Cognitive Behavioral Skills Template** (Session 2, Appendix A) prepared.

- Review the goal, behavior dimension, and E/RP steps that were part of the gradual exposure. Reflect on the steps written on the **Stepping It Up: Completing My Exposures** sheet for targeted OCBs. Examine whether steps need to be adjusted. You can gauge this by looking at the progress (checkmarks) for exposures and colored circles indicating the children engaged in their replacement behaviors. If very little is filled in, explore the understanding of components, child motivation, feasibility of working on exposures, and other relevant variables. Modify as needed to make it feasible for the child and caregivers.

- Using the completed **Stepping It Up: Completing My Exposures** sheet, have the child review the coping techniques they wrote down. If helpful, turn to the coping techniques written down and review the types of coping techniques checked off or preferred by the child. Here are the four types of coping techniques:

  - *Believing in Myself: What I Can Do and Say to OCB*
  - *My Toolbox*
  - *Other Things I Need or Like*
  - *Thinking Differently and Outsmarting OCB*

- Note that the **Functional Behavior Assessment and Intervention (FBAI) Summary Form** (which supports the **Other Things I Need or Like** activity) will be reviewed in the Caregiver Module.

- Use the completed **Stepping It Up: Completing My Exposures** sheet and Session 4 worksheets on coping techniques for OCB #2 to talk about what worked from the child and caregiver's views. Can existing components be expanded on? Are there other coping techniques that could be used? Have the child fill in their coping techniques on the new **Stepping It Up: Completing My Exposures** sheet for what they will do and say to boss back OCB this week.

- Emphasize that coping techniques should be practiced during and/or after completing E/RP steps (and coloring in the circles). Implementing coping techniques (and their timing) will be worked on in Caregiver Module 5 to support intervention for current and future OCBs. In our experience, knowing when and how to be flexible with the use of coping techniques is sometimes a challenge for caregivers and children.

- Last, fill out the rewards by referring to the completed **Rewarding Yourself** and **Small and Big Rewards** worksheets or choosing from the options on the completed **Stepping It Up: Completing My Exposures** sheet from last week. Explore what the children liked and if they received the reward the same day as completing the exposure. Brainstorm preferred items to add in based on their current interests.

Therapist Reflection on Challenges

- Overall, we suggest that you examine whether challenges are related to incorrect or little use of strategies or other variables. If challenges are related to the incorrect use of strategies, model and practice as appropriate. If challenges are related to limited use of strategies, does response effort need to be reduced or the program intensity adjusted?
- Attend to whether new thoughts surrounding the compulsion have been identified. You could also probe for additional thoughts as part of reviewing the **Thinking Differently and Outsmarting OCB** activity. Additional work in the cognitive restructuring area may be beneficial (even in a protracted fashion).
- Note setting events and antecedents that children and youth discuss, as this will help them better understand the OCB and the progress made.

Note: At this point, children will complete Break and Snack (10 Min.) and Social Skills Activity: Freestyle Building (15 Min.) while Caregivers complete Caregiver Module 5: Functional Behavior Assessment and FBAI: Special Topic on Addressing Dual Functions (25 Min.)

Break and Snack

You may continue to offer snacks from the **Reinforcer Checklist** (Chapter 1, Appendix B). Depending on your policies, snacks may be prepared ahead of time, or caregivers may be asked to bring them in.

Allow this break period to be child-directed (e.g., a child may want to draw or attempt to initiate a game with you). You can capitalize on this time to build rapport with the children or facilitate rapport building within the group. If helpful, use a timer and give children reminders of the time remaining.

You may use this time to observe OCBs or contrive situations to collect descriptive data (if possible) using the **ABC Narrative Form** (Chapter 3, Appendix B) or you may use one of your own.

Social Skills Activity: Freestyle Building

Freestyle Building requires children to work together to re-create an image using building blocks (e.g., LEGO®). This is an intermediate social skill activity (see Chapter 4 for further details).

Instructions: Have the children get into pairs (Note: it may be help-ful to have children with similar skill levels paired with one another). Give each pair a bag of construction materials and a picture. Next, tell the group they will be working together to re-create the picture using the construction materials they've been given. For children that build quickly, provide them with more complex pictures or multiple pictures to re-create. Once everyone is finished, encourage each pair to share their structures with the group. After each pair has shared their struc-ture, encourage the group to congratulate them and share what they liked about their structure.

In a one-on-one setting, the child can complete the activity indepen-dently and then share what they created. See Chapter 4 for additional modifications.

Examining Quality of Life

Using the **Quality of Life** activity in the workbook, review the sample of Ally (the girl who wrote down her favorite things and people in the circle). Then, point out the words stuck on top of her favorite things: these are Ally's compulsions. Explain how the *compulsions cover up a lot of Ally's favorite things and people. Her compulsions are covering up many of her favorite things, and they are getting in the way of her being able to do them and spend time with her family and friends.* Mention that *OCBs take up a lot of time, affecting Ally's quality of life or the hap-piness she feels daily. This is why Ally and YOU are working so hard to outsmart OCB!*

Turn to the next page, where you will see a blank circle. Ask the children to do the same thing that Ally did. First, write out or draw their favorite things and people. Then, have the children place their compul-sions on top of their "fun things" inside the circle. They can do this by writing their compulsions on paper, cutting them out, and taping them, or using miniature sticky notes.

Explain to the children that these circles represent Quality of Life and will be revisited as sessions progress. When revisiting the Quality of Life circle, have them remove compulsions that they "beat" or no longer have the urge to do to reveal their preferred items or activities underneath.

While doing this exercise, you may choose to refer to the **Operational Definitions and Interference Form** (Chapter 2, Appendix C). Comment on the different compulsions and their current level of interference (e.g., time spent rearranging stuffed animals if they were moved). You can also discuss the level of distress each one causes if the child isn't able to perform the compulsion (e.g., a child lines up stuffed animals, but the caregiver doesn't attempt to move them because of the history of distress). This allows you to examine changes in the level of interference from the initial assessment to this point in treatment. This information can also be used for programming in Session 6.

Individualized Intervention for OCB #3 and Homework

If not moving on to OCB #3, review previous OCBs as needed.

Refer to your completed **Cognitive Behavioral Skills Template** (Session 2, Appendix A) for OCB #3. Have children complete the **OCB News** for the third OCB. Children are becoming familiar with the different types of coping techniques, but because it is still a new OCB to address, it is suggested that you go through each worksheet in the workbook for Session 5 with the new OCB. In our experience, exposure often aided in children choosing new techniques. Creativity and confidence blossomed! For Session 5, continue structured programming and provide as much assistance as needed. You will likely still be guiding the child and caregiver through these activities. Fade your guidance for the caregiver and have the child take on increasingly more responsibility. Now that you are familiar with the coping techniques, each of the sections and relevant coping techniques will be reviewed briefly. Refer to previous sessions for more details.

Believing in Myself: What I Can Do and Say to OCB

Children and youth are now familiar with bossing back statements and statements communicating acceptance of OCB's presence. For the third OCB, you will begin with the activity **Believing in Myself: What I Can Do and Say to OCB** in the workbook. At this point, if they haven't already done so, children will begin to complete this section independently. Encourage the child to say the statements aloud (if comfortable), picture themselves bossing back OCB, and engage in role-play. Emphasize that the more they practice, the easier it will be to do the coping techniques when they are anxious.

My Toolbox

Review the **My Toolbox** activity and the coping strategies (with pictures). Continue to individualize techniques to the OCBs you are targeting. You likely have the child's favorite strategies on your **Cognitive Behavioral Skills Template** but think about the OCB and what is most applicable.

For example, if the OCB involves vocally asking for reassurance, a technique that involves a vocal response (e.g., counting from 1–10, breathing) may be beneficial.

At this point, you may begin to look for patterns in what worked and did not work for the first two OCBs. What seems to consistently be a good coping strategy? Can you build on previous techniques or look at new techniques listed that would act as a replacement behavior? Again, choose one or two techniques to focus on for the third OCB. Have the caregiver practice prompting, modeling, and providing praise to the child (as practiced in the behavior skills training in this session's Caregiver Module).

Other Things I Need or Like

Referring to the **Functional Behavior Assessment and Intervention (FBAI) Summary Form,** complete the **Other Things I Need or Like** activity. Discuss how this can be incorporated into treatment, building on today's Caregiver Module. The caregiver has now participated in multiple modules on functions of behavior, allowing you to increase their responsibility for leading this activity and providing input on function-based coping techniques. Provide prompting and feedback as needed. In the Caregiver Module for this session, we reviewed function-based interventions that combine multiple functions and when to implement the replacement behaviors (e.g., during and/or after an exposure step).

Thinking Differently and Outsmarting My OCB

Thinking Differently and Outsmarting My OCB is the final activity. See Chapter 1, Thinking Differently: Cognitive Restructuring for a more detailed description of cognitive restructuring and self-talk. You may attempt to restructure or reframe thoughts if appropriate and if the child's cognitive and developmental profile allows for this. Many children often have a difficult time articulating the obsession or thoughts and physiological sensations that precede compulsions. However, depending on the OCB, you may be able to do *some* cognitive restructuring and reframing of thoughts especially if the child becomes more aware and comfortable talking about them. Session 3 offers additional examples that may be suitable for the child you are working with and the OCB.

For children who do not have a thought or have a partial thought that would be difficult to work with, you may move to the part of the worksheet on **Outsmarting my OCB.** See Sessions 3 and 4 for more details on this activity and examples.

Rewarding Yourself

Have the child turn to the **Rewarding Yourself** activities in the workbook. Explain to children that they will write daily rewards on their homework sheet to earn when they're being brave and bossing back OCB. Try to make the connection between the rewards and completing their exposures (and using their coping techniques) each day for them.

The child does not need to fill out all five rewards. Come up with a few and then move on to the next page. Immediate reinforcement is better than delayed reinforcement. Therefore, children will choose daily rewards for completing exposures. Explain to the caregiver and child that many of the rewards should be small rewards that can be delivered each day.

Small and Big Rewards

Given the focus on small rewards on the **Rewarding Yourself** sheet, you may want to encourage children to copy what they have already generated. If you have generated sufficient information in the **Rewarding Yourself** activity, you may choose to skip this sheet. You can refer to this sheet when completing the **Stepping It Up: Completing My Exposures** homework to identify small rewards for daily practice and large rewards for sustained success.

Completing E/RP Worksheet for OCB #3

Explain to the child that it is now time to complete their homework sheet called **Stepping It Up and Completing My Exposures**.

1. Turn to the blank **Stepping It Up and Completing My Exposures** workbook sheet. Review the components if needed. Have the child or caregiver write out the goal.
2. Determine the behavior dimension. Refer to your **Cognitive Behavioral Skills Template** (Session 2, Appendix A) if needed. Write out the daily exposures.
3. List coping techniques. Have the child review the Cognitive Behavior Skills Training sheets as necessary.
4. Refer to the functional behavior assessment and intervention reviewed in Caregiver Module 5 as you complete the **Stepping It Up and Completing My Exposures**.
5. Review instructions on checking circles when completing exposures and coloring in circles when using coping techniques with the child

and caregiver. Tell children and caregivers that coping techniques should be used during and/or after exposures. Given the practice in Caregiver Module 5, caregivers might lead this piece. When at desired levels, coping techniques may be initially needed but then should not be required by the child.

6. The final step is choosing rewards. Have the child refer back to their **Rewarding Yourself** and **Small and Big Rewards** workbook sheets to choose daily rewards. It is optional to have a weekly reward.

Token Exchange and Goodbyes

Complete the token exchange and have the children say goodbye to one another.

Caregiver Module 5: Functional Behavior Assessment and FBAI: Special Topic on Addressing Dual Functions

Review and Introduction

Distribute new **Caregiver Weekly Data Forms** (Chapter 2, Appendix E). Let caregivers know to bring forward issues or challenges when tackling OCBs, or any new OCBs that arise.

Tell the caregivers that this week's module will focus on continuing to build their skills around interpreting their child's completed FBAI summary chart and function-based strategies. We will also focus on replacement behaviors and when it is best for the child to implement them (e.g., during and/or after the exposure step is completed).

Instruction

The first goal is to ensure caregivers are comfortable with their child's FBAI and implementing function-based interventions. Because this is the halfway point, you'll want to review function-based strategies before moving on to E/RP. For the completed FBAI, let caregivers know that this step can be complex when targeting multiple OCBs, so we want to give them ample practice. When treatment is done, these function-based interventions may be used if/when OCBs with similar functions arise (reviewed during Relapse Prevention in Caregiver Modules 7 to 9).

The second goal is for caregivers to become comfortable knowing when to implement function-based strategies and replacement behaviors (e.g., during and/or after exposure steps).

The third goal is to help caregivers understand if/when they can combine function-based interventions. Let caregivers know that as they become more knowledgeable about addressing multiple functions, they may not need to implement every strategy separately. Instead, they may be able to combine strategies (e.g., providing attention contingent on the child participating in deep breathing exercises during gradual exposure steps), as long as both functions are being addressed.

Not all OCBs will be maintained by multiple functions. If this has been identified in your assessments, let the caregiver know the aforementioned point will not apply to them.

Modeling

Show caregivers when to implement their child's function-based interventions (see FBAI Summary Chart; Session 2, Appendix C). Have the caregiver or a therapist act as the child as you demonstrate when to implement the interventions.

An example of what this demonstration could look like has been provided below. In your demonstration, it is likely best to replace this templated example with the child's OCBs and function-based interventions.

Example: A child engages in reassurance-seeking questions that cause significant distress if not answered and often have a secondary attention function. It is sometimes challenging to know when to implement the coping techniques (e.g., during and/or after the exposure step). Here are examples of when to implement function-based strategies and how you may combine function-based strategies:

- When the child is not seeking reassurance, encourage the child to use coping strategies during their regular routine (e.g., if the child is showing signs of mild anxiety or distress, this would be a good time to practice a deep breathing exercise).
- If the child is completing their exposure step (e.g., asking a maximum of five reassurance-seeking questions) and in the midst of question-asking, begins to show signs of distress (e.g., heavy breathing, crying), encourage them to engage in their function-based strategy, such as deep breathing exercises and provide social attention (e.g., praise or a high-five) for doing so.
- After the child has engaged in reassurance seeking, you may redirect them to a conversation around a preferred topic (see Reinforcer Assessment in Chapter 1). Reinforce the child for engaging in replacement/alternative behaviors (e.g., using "bossing back" statements, doing karate movements in OCB's presence) and provide praise for engaging in these replacement behaviors. The latter example shows a way to address both functions (escape from anxiety and access to attention).

Rehearsal

If time permits and the caregivers want the opportunity to practice, support them in taking the lead on the intervention. In group therapy, this can be done one at a time or by dividing caregivers into pairs (e.g., one caregiver can pretend to be the child while the other implements the intervention, and then the roles can be reversed).

If rehearsal isn't possible, tell the caregiver that this will be reviewed thoroughly during individual programming for OCBs later in the session.

Feedback

Provide positive and specific praise when the caregiver demonstrates the intervention correctly (e.g., "You did a great job redirecting to that coping technique and providing attention!") and corrective feedback for incorrect/incomplete components (e.g., "Next time, let's redirect [Child's name] when they begin to whimper instead of waiting for them to scream.")

Scheduling Follow-Up Meetings

Review the **Functional Behavior Assessment and Intervention (FBAI) Summary Form** (Session 2, Appendix C) for the new OCB. If needed, continue to review the completed FBAI for the OCB during individualized programming. Take a few minutes to schedule follow-up meetings with caregivers to complete the functional behavior assessments for the next OCB (see Chapter 3 for details). Finalize which OCBs will be the focus of the upcoming session.

Chapter 11

Session 6

Relapse Prevention and Introducing More Flexibility With OCBs

Materials

- Children's Workbook
- Flipchart/Whiteboard
- Token Board (Session 1, Appendix A)
- Tokens and grab bag of preferred items
- Activities/food items for break/snack
- ABC Narrative Form (Chapter 3, Appendix B)
- Reinforcer Checklist (Chapter 1, Appendix B)
- Cognitive Behavioral Skills Template (Session 2, Appendix A)
- Building Our Greeting Bank materials, two masking tape ladders created on the floor (one ladder for every two children)
- Building Buddies construction materials (e.g., building blocks, LEGO®) and pictures of different structures the children will build
- Blank Caregiver Weekly Data Form (Chapter 2, Appendix E)

Session Outline

- Homework Review (15 Min.)
- Social Skills Activity: Building our Greeting Bank (15 Min.)
- Review of Previous Work on OCBs and Further Programming (25 Min.)
- Break and Snack (10 Min.)
- Social Skills Activity: Building Buddies (15 Min.)
- Individualized Intervention for OCB #4 and Possibly OCB #5 and Homework (35 Min.)
- Token Exchange and Goodbyes (5 Min.)
- Caregiver Module 6: Exposure and Response Prevention: Choosing E/RP Steps (25 Min.) – To take place during Break and Snack, and Building Buddies

DOI: 10.4324/9781003410126-11

Pre-Session Checklist

- Arrange the environment (e.g., seating) as you feel appropriate.
- You may continue to outline the session activities on a whiteboard or flipchart.
- Have child **Token Boards** ready with prosocial behaviors written on them. Vary tokens to depict preferred pictures or stickers to maintain interest.
- Complete the **Cognitive Behavioral Skills Template** (Session 2, Appendix A) for the next target OCBs.
- Prepare new **Caregiver Weekly Data Forms** (Chapter 2, Appendix E).
- Complete the **Functional Behavior Assessment and Intervention (FBAI) Summary Form** (based on functional behavior assessment completed) for the next target OCBs (Session 2, Appendix C).

Session Implementation

Homework Review

Use the first few minutes to collect **Caregiver Weekly Data Forms** (Chapter 2, Appendix E). Review today's schedule and hand out the **Token Boards** (Session 1, Appendix A) with prosocial behaviors written on them for today's session.

Have children give a brief review of progress with their multiple OCBs. Ask caregivers to continue to participate as appropriate. Leading prompts may be given to the children, *"Talk about something that you are proud of,"* or *"Name something that went well this week"* or *"What coping techniques did you use, and were they helpful or not?"* Encourage children to become increasingly independent and add more detail in vocalizing their experiences, recognizing their cognitive, developmental, and socio-emotional profile (see Concrete Learners and Adaptations in Chapter 1, for greater detail).

Ask children to turn to the **Mapping OCB** sheet from Session 2. Using the stimulus map, the **Caregiver Weekly Data Forms** (Chapter 2, Appendix E), and the completed **Stepping It Up: Completing My Exposures** sheets, discuss progress and obstacles with the targeted OCBs. Examine what OCBs can be tackled from the same response class (e.g., two types of ordering and arranging) as well as the more resistant OCBs. Use this time to discuss possible target OCBs for Session 7 and whether a functional behavior assessment should be completed for the next session. This should be discussed with caregivers further in Caregiver Module 6.

Ask the child, *Should [Targeted OCBs] be moved on the stimulus map or do they need to be worked on a little bit more?* Assist the child or youth in making this decision and emphasize that some OCBs take more time than others and move a bit slower to the Me Zone. Usually, by Session 6, some OCBs have moved towards the Me Zone (see definitions of zones in Session 2 if you need a brief review). You may also refer to our definitions of minimal and good progress in helping the child to decide whether the compulsion moves over on the stimulus map to be closer to the Me Zone. Some OCBs may move back and forth between zones if re-emergence occurs.

Continue to discuss the interference of OCBs and how they can impact the quality of life for themselves and their family members. This may increase motivation to continue to engage in treatment and reinforce the need to learn the coping techniques to tackle OCBs when they arise. You may refer to the **Quality of Life** exercise from Session 5. Some children may be able to remove an OCB from their **Quality of Life** exercise that has shown progress since the last session.

Suggested Criteria for Moving to the Next OCBs

Use the data (**Caregiver Weekly Data Forms**, stimulus map, **Stepping It Up: Completing My Exposures** sheets) and a discussion with the caregiver and child to decide whether to program for additional OCBs in this session. Over one week, if progress is being made, you should see some movement toward desired levels on the caregiver rating sheet for individual OCBs (e.g., a rating of five to a rating of three over several days). Also, the child should show increased fluency in using the coping techniques and indicate some success in resisting OCB (which would be indicated by several successful attempts on E/RP steps and using coping techniques). The stimulus map can be used for discussion and assessing progress.

1. Minimal Progress: If the criteria are not met, the team (child, caregiver, therapist) may make the joint decision to continue working on the same OCBs for the following week. You may now be at the point where you are reviewing progress for two OCBs, with one OCB at the desired levels. If the child has made minimal progress on both OCBs or re-emergence has occurred, you may consider pausing here and modifying intervention components as appropriate.
2. Good Progress: If the child has continued to make good progress on the second OCB and it has remained at desired levels (with no need for the use of coping techniques) for at least one week, discontinue

data collection as you did for the first OCB. If the child has also made good progress with the third OCB and the urge to complete it is gone (as evidenced by it being at desired levels for most days with no need for coping techniques), you may discontinue data collection. One week is usually not enough. It will be more likely that the child made some progress, but you encourage continued work on OCB #3 to ensure the urge is completely gone (see case of handwashing described in Session 3). Review and modify the intervention (if necessary) and then fill out another **Stepping It Up: Completing My Exposures** worksheet.

Encourage generalization to other stimuli, settings, and people as appropriate. For OCBs in the same response class (e.g., sitting in the same seat in the car and home) that continue to result in anxiety or distress, an additional individual program plan may be added. For example, a need to sit in the same seat in the car may require a similar but slightly varied treatment plan than sitting in the same seat at the kitchen table. Use your discretion as to whether you add this as the target OCB or program for an additional unrelated OCB.

After the break and Caregiver Module, you will develop a new individualized treatment plan for OCB #4 and possibly OCB #5 on the **Stepping It Up: Completing My Exposures** worksheet. If not moving on, you can discuss the previous OCBs and review coping techniques.

Box 11.1   Tackling the Toughies

As children develop increased familiarity and fluency with functional behavior-based cognitive behavioral therapy (Fb-CBT) components, you may consider adding a more resistant or tough OCB that is causing considerable interference. We have found that adding these at the proper time points with additional strategies to support treatment, such as breaking it down into smaller steps and having several weeks to troubleshoot, is helpful for the child and family. Sometimes it is worth tackling fewer OCBs but ensuring you program for the more troublesome ones. You never want to leave a "toughie" for the child and caregiver to tackle post-treatment. Sometimes these OCBs take longer than three or four weeks, but you can work intensively with the family to develop a solid intervention plan. Booster sessions are also an option which will be discussed in Session 8.

Box 11.2   Adding OCBs

Adding new OCBs has been put into a concrete framework for you to work with (see Table 5.1, Chapter 5). We realize that with variables like re-emergence, motivation, family dynamics, and some OCBs being more difficult than others, you may deviate from this framework. We found it helpful to have a standard framework to use in our work to keep on track. You may choose to use it as a guide, especially as you start working on more difficult OCBs or what we labeled "tackling the toughies."

Social Skills Activity: Building Our Greeting Bank

Building Our Greeting Bank involves children working together to think of a variety of ways to greet others. This is an intermediate social skill activity (see Chapter 4 for further details).

Instructions: Bring the children over to the two masking tape ladders on the floor (there should be one ladder for every two children). Inform children to find a friend/partner to work with. For children who are reluctant, encourage/facilitate the initiation to choose a partner. Describe that the objective of the game is to stand on opposite sides of the greeting ladder and reach the center to collect pretend "money" for their greeting bank. Describe how this "money" can "buy" help when you and your partner are unsure of a way to show that you are proud of each other. Provide each pair with starter "money" (relative to the cost of help and how many ladder spaces there are). Provide examples of how the children can earn more "money". The children can only move forward one spot once each partner has practiced showing their friend one way they are proud of them. For example, each child can hop one step of the ladder when they have given their friend a thumbs up, or each child can hop one step of the ladder when they have yelled "Great work." Have a therapist and another adult model the same examples that were just described. On the third rung have the pair "buy" help from another adult. Any remaining "money" can be exchanged for a token which they can put on their token board. Tell the children to start climbing and building their greeting bank. Encourage the children to use the things learned today next time they are proud of their friend.

In a one-on-one setting, the therapist and/or caregivers can participate in creating the greetings with the child. See Chapter 4 for additional modifications.

Review of Previous Work on OCBs and Further Programming

Take this time to review the previous work on OCBs and continue programming as needed. Now that you are familiar with our suggested steps, we list them below for your quick review (refer to Sessions 4 and 5 if you need more detail). At this point, you may need to program for OCBs that have re-emerged.

- Review the completed **Stepping It Up: Completing My Exposures** sheet and begin working on a new **Stepping It Up: Completing My Exposures** in the workbook. Have your **Cognitive Behavioral Skills Template** (Session 2, Appendix A) prepared. If OCBs have re-emerged, you may need to prepare additional copies of blank **Stepping It Up: Completing My Exposures** sheets.
- Review the goal, behavior dimension, and exposure and response prevention steps that were part of the gradual exposure. Reflect on the steps written on the **Stepping It Up: Completing My Exposures** sheet for targeted OCBs.
- Using the completed **Stepping It Up: Completing My Exposures** sheets, have the child review the coping techniques they wrote down. Here are the four types of coping techniques:
  - *Believing in Myself: What I Can Do and Say to OCB*
  - *My Toolbox*
  - *Other Things I Need or Like*
  - *Thinking Differently and Outsmarting OCB*
- Review the **Functional Behavior Assessment and Intervention (FBAI) Summary Form** distributed in the Caregiver Module as appropriate.
- Use the completed **Stepping It Up: Completing My Exposures** sheets, and previously completed sheets on coping techniques to decide as a team what should be added.
- Emphasize that coping techniques should be practiced during and/or after completing exposure and response prevention steps (and coloring in the circles).
- Last, fill out the rewards by referring to the completed **Rewarding Yourself** and **Small and Big Rewards** worksheets or choosing from the options on the completed **Stepping It Up: Completing My Exposures** sheet from last week.

Note: At this point, children will complete Break and Snack (10 Min.) and Social Skills Activity: Building Buddies (15 Min.) while Caregivers

complete Caregiver Module 6: Exposure and Response Prevention: Choosing E/RP Steps (25 Min.)

Break and Snack

You may continue to offer snacks from the **Reinforcer Checklist** (Chapter 1, Appendix B). Depending on your policies, snacks may be prepared ahead of time or caregivers may be asked to bring in snacks.

Allow this break period to be child-directed (e.g., a child may want to draw or attempt to initiate a game with you). You can capitalize on this time to build rapport with the children or facilitate rapport building within the group. If helpful, use a timer and give children reminders of the time remaining.

You may use this time to observe OCBs or contrive situations to collect descriptive data (if possible) using the **ABC Narrative Form** (Chapter 3, Appendix B) or you may use one of your own.

Social Skills Activity: Building Buddies

Building Buddies requires children to work together to construct a building. This is an intermediate social skill activity (see Chapter 4 for further details).

Instructions: Ask the children to reflect on the Freestyle Building activity. Ask them what they built in that activity – this can help them think of similar things to build during this activity. Have the children get into groups of three (Note: it may be helpful to have children with similar skill levels grouped). Let the group know that each child will have a special role in their small groups – Engineer, Supplier, and Builder. Model each of these three roles (e.g., sharing ideas as the Engineer, distributing the blocks as the Supplier, and putting pieces together as the Builder). Give each group a bag of building blocks (e.g., LEGO®) and name tags to remind each child of their role. Tell the children they can start creating a building of their choice. When everyone is finished, encourage each triad to share their buildings with the group. After each triad has shared their building, encourage the group to congratulate them and share what they liked about their building.

In a one-on-one setting, the child can be given the choice of completing the activity on their own, and then sharing what they created. See Chapter 4 for additional modifications.

Individualized Intervention for OCB #4 and Possibly OCB #5 and Homework

If not moving on to OCB #4, review previous OCBs as needed.

Refer to your completed **Cognitive Behavioral Skills Template** (Session 2, Appendix A) for OCB #4 and possibly #5. Have children complete the **OCB News** for the fourth and possibly fifth OCB. You may offer more flexibility to the child in picking and choosing which coping technique worksheets to attend to. Likely, you will still be guiding the child and caregiver through choosing coping techniques to add to the **Stepping It Up: Completing My Exposures** sheet. Continue to transfer responsibility to the caregiver and have them take on more independently. Continue to have the child take on increasingly more tasks as they progress through Sessions 6 to 9.

Believing in Myself: What I Can Do and Say to OCB

Children and youth are now familiar with bossing back statements and statements communicating acceptance of OCB's presence. For the fourth and possibly fifth OCB, encourage children to complete the activity independently.

Discussion of My Toolbox

Review the **My Toolbox** activity and the coping strategies (with pictures) as appropriate. Continue to individualize techniques to the OCBs you are targeting. You likely have the child's "favorite" strategies on your **Cognitive Behavioral Skills Template**. In Session 5, we discussed matching a vocal compulsion with a suitable coping strategy and considering the social function. For this session, you may want to spend some extra time brainstorming multiple techniques for a more resistant OCB with the child and caregiver.

Other Things I Need or Like

Referring to the **Functional Behavior Assessment and Intervention (FBAI) Summary Form,** complete the **Other Things I Need or Like** activity and ensure that function-based strategies are discussed and included in the programming. The caregiver has now participated in multiple modules on functions of behavior, allowing you to increase their responsibility for leading this activity and providing input on function-based coping techniques. Provide prompting and feedback as needed.

Thinking Differently and Outsmarting My OCB

Thinking Differently and Outsmarting My OCB is the final activity. See Chapter 1, Thinking Differently: Cognitive Restructuring for a more detailed description of cognitive restructuring and self-talk. By Session 6, we hope that children and youth have developed some reliable coping techniques and are becoming increasingly fluent in choosing and utilizing them while completing exposure steps. Children who can engage in cognitive restructuring can start to have some independence in challenging and reframing thoughts with prompts from the therapist.

For children who do not have a thought or perhaps have a partial thought that would be difficult to work with, you may move to the part of the worksheet on **Outsmarting my OCB.**

Rewarding Yourself

Have the child turn to the **Rewarding Yourself** activities in the workbook. Explain to children that they will write daily rewards on their homework sheet to earn when they're being brave and bossing back OCB. Try to make the connection for them between the rewards and completing their exposures (and using their coping techniques) each day.

The child does not need to fill out all five rewards. Come up with a few and then move on to the next page. Immediate reinforcement is better than delayed reinforcement. Therefore, children will choose daily rewards for completing exposures. Explain to the caregiver and child that many of the rewards should be small rewards that can be delivered each day.

Small and Big Rewards

Given the focus on small rewards on the **Rewarding Yourself** sheet, you may want to encourage children to copy what they have already generated. If you have generated sufficient information in the **Rewarding Yourself** activity, you may choose to skip this sheet. You can refer to this sheet when completing the **Stepping It Up: Completing My Exposures** homework to identify small rewards for daily practice and large rewards for sustained success.

Completing E/RP Worksheet for OCB #4 and Possibly OCB #5

Explain to the child that it is now time to complete their homework sheet called **Stepping It Up and Completing My Exposures**.

1. Turn to the blank **Stepping It Up and Completing My Exposures** workbook sheet. Review the components if needed. Have the child or caregiver write out the goal.
2. Determine the behavior dimension. Refer to your **Cognitive Behavioral Skills Template** (Session 2, Appendix A) if needed. Write out the daily exposures. Given this was the training topic for today's Caregiver Module, encourage the caregiver to try to take the lead on this piece.
3. List coping techniques. Have the child review the Cognitive Behavior Skills Training sheets as necessary.
4. Refer to the functional behavior assessment and intervention reviewed in Caregiver Module 6 as you complete the **Stepping It Up and Completing My Exposures**.
5. Review instructions on checking circles when completing exposures and coloring in circles when using coping techniques with the child and caregiver. Tell children and caregivers that coping techniques should be used during and/or after exposures. Caregivers might begin to lead this piece. When at desired levels, coping techniques may be initially needed but then should not be required by the child.
6. The final step is choosing rewards. Have the child refer back to their **Rewarding Yourself** and **Small and Big Rewards** workbook sheets to choose daily rewards. It is optional to have a weekly reward.

Token Exchange and Goodbyes

Complete the token exchange and have the children say goodbye to one another.

Caregiver Module 6: Exposure and Response Prevention: Choosing E/RP Steps

Review and Introduction

Distribute new **Caregiver Weekly Data Forms** (Chapter 2, Appendix E). Let caregivers know to bring forward issues or challenges when tackling OCBs, or any new OCBs that arise.

Tell the caregivers that this week's module will focus on continuing to build their skills around filling out their child's **Stepping It Up and Completing My Exposure** worksheet for new OCBs, which includes identifying the dimensions of behaviors and formulating exposure steps.

Instruction

Briefly explain the dimensions of behavior. Given limited time, focus on the most common dimensions unless another dimension would be more appropriate for the caregiver and child. Examples include:

- Frequency: How many times a behavior happens (e.g., the child arranges stuffed animals ten times).
- Duration: How long a behavior lasts (e.g., the child engages in handwashing for ten minutes).
- Intensity: The strength of the behavior (e.g., the child must forcefully slam shut every door he walks through).
- Latency: How long it takes for the behavior to begin (e.g., the child moves a toy back into place two minutes after it was moved out of place).
- Topography: The way the behavior looks (e.g., the child performs a routine by completing ten steps in a certain order).

See Table 1.1 in Chapter 1 for more details and additional examples.

Next, provide each caregiver with a blank copy of the **Stepping It Up and Completing My Exposure** worksheet (Children's Workbook). Briefly reiterate the purpose of each component of the worksheet:

- Goal: The goal your child is aiming to achieve during treatment (e.g., reducing the OCB to a desired level).
- Exposure Steps: Each step represents a gradual progression from the child's current level of OCB to their desired goal. Using a chosen topography to measure the behavior (e.g., frequency), each step should represent an achievable improvement in the child's OCB

(e.g., progressing from engaging in 20 reassurance-seeking questions to 15 to 10, and so on). Think of each step as a short-term or "mini" goal to help the child reach their long-term or desired goal.

Let caregivers know that the reinforcement component of the **Stepping It Up and Completing My Exposure** worksheet will be discussed in future Caregiver Modules. Ask caregivers to bring the worksheets they complete this week to Caregiver Module 7 or ask them to hand it in at the end of the session so you can redistribute them next week.

Modeling

Show caregivers how to fill out a **Stepping It Up and Completing My Exposure** worksheet with the samples provided. Offer all three examples and allow caregivers to choose which example best fits their child's own OCB.

- Goal #1: Decreasing handwashing duration (Children's Workbook)
    - Progression toward the goal is represented by gradually decreasing the duration of handwashing from seven minutes to one minute.
- Goal #2: Decreasing asking for reassurance (Session 3, Appendix A)
    - Progression toward the goal is represented by gradually reducing the frequency of questions asked from five to none (and instead pointing to a written statement).
- Goal #3: Mixing up the order of stuffed animals (Session 3, Appendix B)
    - Progression toward the goal is represented by gradually changing the topography (e.g., tolerating one stuffed animal moved out of order to tolerating three or more stuffed animals moved out of order).

Rehearsal

Work together with caregivers to identify their child's behavior dimension and then complete the exposure steps portion of their child's **Stepping It Up and Completing My Exposure** worksheet. If you run out of time, this can be done during the individual programming portion of today's session.

Feedback

Provide positive and specific praise when the caregiver completes a portion of the worksheet correctly (e.g., "That's a great progression!") and corrective feedback for incorrect/incomplete components (e.g., "Those two steps might be too challenging for [Child's name]. Let's think of an intermediate step to add in between them.")

Scheduling Follow-Up Meetings

Review the **Functional Behavior Assessment and Intervention (FBAI) Summary Form** (Session 2, Appendix C) for the new OCB. If needed, continue to review the completed FBAI for the OCBs during individualized programming. Take a few minutes to schedule follow-up meetings with caregivers to complete the functional behavior assessments for the next OCBs (see Chapter 3 for details). Finalize which OCBs will be the focus of the upcoming session.

Chapter 12

Session 7

Relapse Prevention, Generalization, and Introducing More Flexibility With OCBs

Materials

- Children's Workbook
- Flipchart/Whiteboard
- Token Board (Session 1, Appendix A)
- Tokens and grab bag of preferred items
- Collect, Pass, Run, and Sort – The Running Relay materials: three sheets of paper, four labeled plastic baskets, three bags, and three sets of grocery item pictures for activity
- Activities/food items for break/snack
- Reinforcer Checklist (Chapter 1, Appendix B)
- ABC Narrative Form (Chapter 3, Appendix B)
- Build and Borrow construction materials (e.g., building blocks, LEGO®) and pictures of different structures the children will build
- Cognitive Behavioral Skills Template (Session 2, Appendix A)
- Blank Caregiver Weekly Data Form (Chapter 2, Appendix E)

Session Outline

- Homework Review (15 Min.)
- Review of Previous Work on OCBs and Further Programming (25 Min.)
- Social Skills Activity: Collect, Pass, Run, and Sort – Running Relay (15 Min.)
- Break and Snack (10 Min.)
- Social Skills Activity: Build and Borrow (15 Min.)
- Individualized Interventions for Multiple Targeted OCBs (35 Min.)
- Token Exchange and Goodbyes (5 Min.)
- Caregiver Module 7: Introduction to Reinforcement (25 Min.) – To take place during Break and Snack, and Build and Borrow

DOI: 10.4324/9781003410126-12

Pre-Session Checklist

- Arrange the environment (e.g., seating) as you feel appropriate.
- You may continue to outline the session activities on a whiteboard or flipchart.
- Have child **Token Boards** ready with prosocial behaviors written on them. Vary tokens to depict preferred pictures or stickers to maintain interest.
- Complete the **Cognitive Behavioral Skills Template** (Session 2, Appendix A) for next target OCBs.
- Prepare new **Caregiver Weekly Data Forms** (Chapter 2, Appendix E).
- Complete the **Functional Behavior Assessment and Intervention (FBAI) Summary Form** (based on functional behavior assessment completed) for next target OCBs (Session 2, Appendix C).

Session Implementation

Homework Review

Use the first few minutes to collect **Caregiver Weekly Data Forms** (Chapter 2, Appendix E). Review today's schedule and hand out the **Token Boards** (Session 1, Appendix A) with prosocial behaviors written on them for today's session. Have children give a brief review of progress with multiple OCBs. Ask caregivers to continue to participate as appropriate. Leading prompts may be given to the children. You may have introduced a more resistant OCB last week, and if so, it likely would be beneficial to ask about this and how it went.

Ask children to turn to the **Mapping OCB** sheet from Session 2. Using the stimulus map, the **Caregiver Weekly Data Forms** (Chapter 2, Appendix E), and the completed **Stepping It Up: Completing My Exposures** sheets, discuss progress and obstacles with target OCBs (including the toughies!). Examine OCBs from the same response class (e.g., two types of ordering and arranging). Suppose you have not observed generalization with behaviors from the same class. In that case, you may try using similar strategies for multiple OCBs in the same class when programming and continue to emphasize practicing coping techniques. Children may also be able to generate strategies more independently. Continued practice and increased independence generating and using coping techniques in the moment will aid in relapse prevention.

At this point, you may choose to become more flexible in the introduction of OCBs. Consider OCBs from similar classes, ones that the child is motivated to work on, and some of the tougher ones that require more intensive programming. If introduced in Sessions 6 and 7, there is plenty of time to modify programming. Use this time to map out remaining OCBs. Also, discuss possible target OCBs for Session 8 and whether a functional behavior assessment (FBA) should be completed for that session. This should be discussed with caregivers further in Caregiver Module 7.

Ask the child, *Should [Targeted OCBs] be moved on the map or do they need to be worked on a little bit more?* Assist the child or youth in making this decision, if needed. Given you may be working on tougher and more resistant OCBs, the child may experience slower movement to the Me Zone. Reiterate to the child that this is expected and that taking small steps is sometimes needed to achieve a larger goal! Continue to discuss the interference of OCBs and how they can impact the quality of life for themselves and their family members. Refer to the **Quality of Life** exercise in Session 5 and encourage children to remove OCBs as appropriate.

Suggested Criteria for Moving to the Next OCBs

Use the data (**Caregiver Weekly Data Forms**, stimulus map, **Stepping It Up: Completing My Exposures** sheets) and a discussion with the caregiver and child to decide whether to program for additional OCBs in this session. Over one week, if progress is being made, you should see some movement toward desired levels on the caregiver rating sheet for individual OCBs (e.g., a rating of five to a rating of three over several days). Also, the child should show increased fluency in using the coping techniques and indicate some success in resisting OCB (which would be indicated by several successful attempts on E/RP steps and using coping techniques). The stimulus map can be used for discussion and assessing progress.

1. Minimal Progress: If the criteria are not met, the team (child, caregiver, therapist) may make the joint decision to continue working on the same OCBs for the following week. You may now be at the point where you are reviewing progress for multiple OCBs. If the child has made minimal progress on OCBs or re-emergence has occurred, you may pause and modify intervention programs as appropriate.
2. Good Progress: If the child has continued to make good progress on the third OCB and it has remained at desired levels (with no need for the use of coping techniques) for at least one week, discontinue data collection. If the child has also made good progress with the fourth

and possibly fifth OCB and the urge to complete them is gone (as evidenced by them being at desired levels for most days with no need for coping techniques), you may discontinue data collection. One week is usually not enough. It will be more likely that the child made some progress, but you encourage continued work on OCBs #4 and #5 to ensure the urge is essentially gone. Review and modify the intervention (if necessary) and then fill out **Stepping It Up: Completing My Exposures** worksheets.

Encourage generalization to other stimuli, settings, and people as appropriate. In Session 6, you may have chosen to add OCBs from the same response class (e.g., sitting on the same seat in the car and home) if generalization did not occur and different program plans were needed. You may introduce OCBs in the same class or consider others that the child is motivated to tackle, including more resistant and interfering OCBs.

After the break and Caregiver Module, you will develop new individualized treatment plans for OCBs on the **Stepping It Up: Completing My Exposures** worksheet.

Box 12.1   Adding OCBs

Adding new OCBs has been put into a concrete framework for you to work with (see Table 5.1, Chapter 5). We realize that with variables like re-emergence, motivation, family dynamics, and some OCBs being more difficult than others, you may deviate from this framework. We found it helpful to have a standard framework to use in our work to keep on track. You may choose to use it as a guide, especially as you start working on more difficult OCBs or what we labeled "tackling the toughies."

Review of Previous Work on OCBs and Further Programming

Take this time to review the previous work on OCBs and continue programming as needed. Now that you are familiar with our suggested steps, we list them briefly for your review (refer to Sessions 4 and 5 if you need more detail). At this point, you may need to program for OCBs that have re-emerged.

- Review the completed **Stepping It Up: Completing My Exposures** sheets and begin working on a new **Stepping It Up: Completing My**

Exposures sheets in the workbook. Have your **Cognitive Behavioral Skills Template** (Session 2, Appendix A) prepared. If OCBs have re-emerged, you may need to prepare additional copies of blank **Stepping It Up: Completing My Exposures** sheets.

- Review the goal, behavior dimension, and exposure and response prevention steps that were part of the gradual exposure. Reflect on the steps written on the **Stepping It Up: Completing My Exposures** worksheet for targeted OCBs.
- Using the completed **Stepping It Up: Completing My Exposures** sheets, have the child review the coping techniques they wrote down. Here are the four types of coping techniques:

  - *Believing in Myself: What I Can Do and Say to OCB*
  - *My Toolbox*
  - *Other Things I Need or Like*
  - *Thinking Differently and Outsmarting OCB*

- Review the **Functional Behavior Assessment and Intervention (FBAI) Summary Form** distributed in the Caregiver Module as appropriate.
- Use the previously completed sheets on coping techniques to decide as a team what should be added.
- Last, fill out the rewards by referring to the completed **Rewarding Yourself** and **Small and Big Rewards** worksheets or choosing from the options on the completed **Stepping It Up: Completing My Exposures** sheet from last week.

Social Skills Activity: Collect, Pass, Run, and Sort – Running Relay

The Collect, Pass, Run, and Sort – Running Relay involves children working together to complete a relay and scavenger hunt. This is an intermediate social skill activity (see Chapter 4 for further details).

Instructions: Place grocery item pictures around the room and mark the floor with prompts for where each child should stand according to their role (e.g., Passer, Runner, Sorter). Each picture corresponds with a corresponding picture in each child's grocery basket. Inform the children to get into groups of three and assign each child one of the three roles. Inform the children that the goal is to collect all the grocery items as a team using their designated roles. If needed, you can model the scavenger hunt. Say *"On your mark, get set, GO!"* to start the race. Prompt the children to encourage one another. Once all items have been retrieved and sorted, have the children switch roles and repeat the activity. If time permits, do this until each child has had a turn playing each of the three roles.

In a one-on-one setting, the therapist and/or caregiver may participate in the relay race with the child, or the child can perform the relay more than once and try to do it in the fastest time. See Chapter 4 for additional modifications.

Note: At this point, children will complete Break and Snack (10 Min.) and Social Skills Activity: Build and Borrow (15 Min.) while Caregivers complete Caregiver Module 7: Introduction to Reinforcement (25 Min.)

Break and Snack

You may continue to offer snacks from the **Reinforcer Checklist** (Chapter 1, Appendix B). Depending on your policies, snacks may be prepared ahead of time, or caregivers may be asked to bring in snacks.

Allow this break period to be child-directed (e.g., a child may want to draw or attempt to initiate a game with you). You can capitalize on this time to build rapport with the children or facilitate rapport building within the group. If helpful, use a timer and give children reminders of the time remaining.

You may use this time to observe OCBs or contrive situations to collect descriptive data (if possible) using the **ABC Narrative Form** (Chapter 3, Appendix B), or you may use one of your own.

Social Skills Activity: Build and Borrow

Build and Borrow requires children to work together to construct a building and communicate with members of other groups. This is an advanced social skill activity (see Chapter 4 for further details) that builds upon the skills the children learned in Building Buddies (Session 6).

Instructions: Have the children get into pairs (Note: it may be helpful to have children with similar skill levels paired with one another). Give each pair a bag of building blocks (e.g., LEGO®) and a picture. Each bag of blocks only contains one style of block (e.g., Pair 1 has the blue blocks, Pair 2 has the red blocks, etc.). Tell the children they will be working in pairs to re-create the picture using the blocks they've been given. Ask the children what they notice about their bags of blocks and what they need to do to re-create their pictures (sharing their blocks with other groups). For children who build quickly, provide them with more complex pictures or multiple pictures to re-create. Once everyone is finished, encourage each pair to share their structures with the group.

After each pair has shared their structure, encourage the group to congratulate them and share what they liked about their structure.

In a one-on-one setting, the child can be given the choice of completing the activity on their own, then sharing what they created, or completing the activity cooperatively with the therapist and/or their caregivers. See Chapter 4 for additional modifications.

Individualized Interventions for Multiple Targeted OCBs

Refer to your completed **Cognitive Behavioral Skills Template** (Session 2, Appendix A). Have children complete the **OCB News** for OCBs where you think this would be helpful. By Week 7, you will continue fading your guidance for the caregiver and having them assume a more independent role in programming. This may vary with the OCB you are targeting (e.g., they may need more guidance with programming for the more resistant OCBs). Have the child take on increasingly more responsibility. See Sessions 3 through 6 for an explanation of the four types of coping techniques: **Believing in Myself: What I Can Do and Say to OCB, My Toolbox, Other Things I Need or Like, Thinking Differently, and Outsmarting OCB**. Complete the **Rewarding Yourself** and **Small and Big Rewards** activities as needed.

Completing E/RP Worksheets for the Multiple Targeted OCBs

Explain to the child that it is now time to complete their homework sheet called **Stepping It Up and Completing My Exposures**. See Sessions 3 through 6 for a detailed explanation of how to complete each of the components. Given Caregiver Module 7 is on Choosing Reinforcers, attempt to have caregivers take a larger role in the selection of reinforcers and programming for OCBs at desired levels and new OCBs.

Token Exchange and Goodbyes

Complete the token exchange and have the children say goodbye to one another. Remind children to bring an item to share next session.

Caregiver Module 7: Introduction to Reinforcement

Review and Introduction

Distribute new **Caregiver Weekly Data Forms** (Chapter 2, Appendix E). Let caregivers know to bring forward issues or challenges when tackling OCBs, or any new OCBs that arise.

Tell the caregivers that this week's module will involve continuing to fill out their child's **Stepping It Up and Completing My Exposures** worksheet for new OCBs and identifying both small and large reinforcers.

Instruction

Remind caregivers what reinforcers are: preferred items, activities, or social interactions given to the child after they engage in behavior that increases the likelihood of that specific behavior happening again in the future. In other words, reinforcers are something the child likes and is willing to "work for."

Explain the difference between small and large reinforcers:

* Small reinforcers: Less expensive, moderately preferred, and readily available items (e.g., ten minutes with a toy or activity, or a favorite person, stickers, or tokens). Small reinforcers are given when children complete the daily exposure steps and/or maintain an OCB at the desirable level (e.g., handwashing was reduced to one minute for one day and it was maintained at that duration for consecutive days in the review week).
* Large reinforcers: More expensive, highly preferred items that may not be as readily available as smaller reinforcers (e.g., one hour with a toy or activity, receiving a larger toy, or an outing). Large reinforcers are given when children complete multiple days of exposure (this can be flexible and should vary based on each child's needs) and/or if the child overcomes a particularly challenging exposure step. For example, tokens (e.g., stickers) can be given daily for the child to exchange for a larger reinforcer (e.g., going to the arcade) at the end of the week.

The types of reinforcers and when they are delivered should be chosen based on each child's needs and the suitability for each family's schedule.

Modeling

Give each caregiver their completed copy of the **Stepping It Up and Completing My Exposures** worksheet from last week. Show caregivers how to fill out the reinforcement portion of the worksheet using one of the samples provided:

- Goal #1: Decreasing handwashing duration (Children's Workbook)

  - Small reinforcers (e.g., the child will receive when they complete the daily exposure steps): ten minutes of iPad time, a milkshake, or a new Pop-It toy.
  - Large reinforcers (e.g., the child will receive when they complete six to seven exposure steps or if the child overcomes a particularly challenging exposure step): Going to see a movie.

- Goal #2: Decreasing asking for reassurance (Session 3, Appendix A)

  - Small reinforcers (e.g., the child will receive when they complete the daily exposure steps): 20 minutes with dad, ice cream, or picking out a snack at the store.
  - Large reinforcers (e.g., the child will receive when they complete six to seven exposure steps or if the child overcomes a particularly challenging exposure step): Going to the beach.

- Goal #3: Mixing up the order of stuffed animals (Session 3, Appendix B)

  - Small reinforcers (e.g., the child will receive when they complete the daily exposure steps): 10 extra minutes of screen time, new coloring sheets, or getting to pick that day's dessert.
  - Large reinforcers (e.g., the child will receive when they complete six to seven exposure steps or if the child overcomes a particularly challenging exposure step): Going to the arcade.

If needed, provide caregivers with a completed copy of their child's **Reinforcer Checklist** (Chapter 1, Appendix B).

Rehearsal

Work with caregivers to help them identify their child's small and large reinforcers for a current OCB. Then, complete the reinforcer portion of their child's **Stepping It Up and Completing My Exposures** worksheet. If you run out of time, this can be done during the individual programming portion of today's session.

Feedback

The caregivers are working on identifying a suitable reinforcer for the first exposure step. Provide positive and specific praise when the caregiver completes a portion of the worksheet correctly (e.g., "That reinforcer is perfect for that exposure step!") and corrective feedback for incorrect/ incomplete components (e.g., "That reinforcer might be a bit too big. What's something smaller you can give [Child's name] instead?").

Scheduling Follow-Up Meetings

Review the **Functional Behavior Assessment and Intervention (FBAI) Summary Form** (Session 2, Appendix C) for the new OCB. If needed, continue to review the completed FBAI for the OCB during individualized programming. Take a few minutes to schedule follow-up meetings with caregivers to complete the FBA for the next OCBs (see Chapter 3 for details). Finalize which OCBs will be the focus of the upcoming session.

Chapter 13

Session 8

Relapse Prevention, Generalization, and Tackling Final OCBs

Materials

- Flipchart/Whiteboard
- Token Board (Session 1, Appendix A)
- Tokens and grab bag of preferred items
- Share-A-Way materials, including personal items from home
- Activities/food items for break/snack
- Reinforcer Checklist (Chapter 1, Appendix B)
- ABC Narrative Form (Chapter 3, Appendix B)
- Picture Prep materials, a camera, and any materials children would like to include in their photos (e.g., costumes, favorite toys, funky hairdos, homemade masks)
- Cognitive Behavioral Skills Template (Session 2, Appendix A)
- Blank Caregiver Weekly Data Form (Chapter 2, Appendix E)

Session Outline

- Homework Review (15 Min.)
- Social Skills Activity: Share-A-Way (15 Min.)
- Review of Previous Work on OCBs and Further Programming (25 Min.)
- Break and Snack (10 Min.)
- Social Skills Activity: Picture Prep (15 Min.)
- Individualized Interventions for the Multiple Targeted OCBs (35 Min.)
- Token Exchange and Goodbyes (5 Min.)
- Caregiver Module 8: Reinforcement Thinning (25 Min.) – To take place during Break and Snack, and Picture Prep

DOI: 10.4324/9781003410126-13

Pre-Session Checklist

- Arrange the environment (e.g., seating) as you feel appropriate.
- You may continue to outline the session activities on a whiteboard or flipchart.
- Have child **Token Boards** ready with prosocial behaviors written on them. Vary tokens to depict preferred pictures or stickers to maintain interest.
- Complete the **Cognitive Behavioral Skills Template** (Session 2, Appendix A) for next target OCBs.
- Prepare new **Caregiver Weekly Data Forms** (Chapter 2, Appendix E).
- Complete the **Functional Behavior Assessment and Intervention (FBAI) Summary Form** (based on functional behavior assessment completed) for next target OCBs (Session 2, Appendix C).

Session Implementation

Homework Review

Use the first few minutes to collect **Caregiver Weekly Data Forms** (Chapter 2, Appendix E). Review today's schedule and hand out the **Token Boards** (Session 1, Appendix A) with prosocial behaviors written on them for today's session. Have children give a brief review of progress with multiple OCBs. Leading prompts to encourage conversation should be offered as needed.

Using the stimulus map, the **Caregiver Weekly Data Forms** (Chapter 2, Appendix E), and the completed **Stepping It Up: Completing My Exposures** sheet, discuss progress and obstacles with target OCBs, including the more complex and resistant ones. Check if generalization has occurred from OCBs in the same or different response classes. Ask the question: *Should your OCBs be moved on the map?* Likely, children will initiate this on their own.

Encourage practice and independence in using coping techniques in the moment to support relapse prevention. You may also have the child look at OCBs in various zones on the stimulus map and discuss setting events (or circumstances that lead to an increased likelihood of OCBs occurring). The child and the caregiver could discuss current and future setting events (e.g., being ill) and how the child may increase the use of coping techniques or ask for a caregiver to participate in resisting the urge to give in to an OCB. Understanding the relationship between OCBs and setting events can aid in relapse prevention. Focus on a few setting events for this session; returning to this topic in Session 9 would likely be helpful.

Discuss what OCBs are left and need to be programmed for in Session 9. In some cases, children and caregivers may want to develop a complete intervention plan for an OCB to work on and discuss post-treatment (e.g., in a booster session). In this case, a functional behavior assessment (FBA) may be scheduled for this coming week, which can be further discussed in Caregiver Module 8.

Suggested Criteria for Moving to the Next OCBs

Use the data (caregiver data sheets, stimulus map, E/RP worksheets) and a discussion with the caregiver and child to decide whether to program for an additional OCB in this session. Over one week, if progress is being made, you should see some movement toward desired levels on the caregiver rating sheet for individual OCBs (e.g., a rating of five to a rating of three over several days). Also, the child should show increased fluency in using the coping techniques and indicate some success in resisting OCB (which would be indicated by several successful attempts on E/RP steps and using coping techniques). The stimulus map can be used for discussion and assessing progress.

1. Minimal Progress: If the criteria are not met, the team (child, caregiver, therapist) may decide jointly to continue working on the same OCBs for the following week.
2. Good Progress: If the child has continued to make good progress on targeted OCBs and has remained at desired levels (with no need for using coping techniques) for at least one week, discontinue data collection. One week is usually not enough. It will be more likely that the child made some progress, but you encourage continued work in the 25-minute "Review of Previous Work on OCBs."

Encourage generalization to other stimuli, settings, and people as appropriate. You may introduce OCBs in the same class or consider others that the child is motivated to tackle, including more resistant and interfering OCBs.

After the break and Caregiver Module, you will develop new individualized treatment plans for OCBs on the **Stepping It Up: Completing My Exposures** worksheet.

Social Skills Activity: Share-A-Way

Share-A-Way involves children sharing information and listening while others share information. This is an advanced social skill activity (see Chapter 4 for further details).

Instructions: Break children into groups of two. Instruct the children to take out their item for sharing. Model appropriate behavior to children by sharing your item first. Prompt the children to begin sharing their item with their partner. Once children have shared with their partner, have the children share with the larger group.

In a one-on-one setting, the child may informally share and discuss their item with the therapist or caregivers. See Chapter 4 for additional modifications.

Review of Previous Work on OCBs and Further Programming

Take this time to review the previous work on OCBs and continue programming as needed. Now that you are familiar with our suggested steps, we list them briefly for your review (refer to Sessions 4 and 5 if you need more details). Have the completed E/RP worksheets and blank E/RP sheets from the Children's Workbook. If OCBs have re-emerged, you may need to photocopy more worksheets.

- Review the completed **Stepping It Up: Completing My Exposures** page and begin working on a new **Stepping It Up: Completing My Exposures** sheet in the workbook. Have your **Cognitive Behavioral Skills Template** (Session 2, Appendix A) prepared.
- Review the goal, behavior dimension, and exposure and response prevention steps that were part of the gradual exposure. Reflect on the steps written on the **Stepping It Up: Completing My Exposures** worksheet for targeted OCBs.
- Using the completed **Stepping It Up: Completing My Exposures** sheets, have the child review the coping techniques they wrote down. Here are the four types of coping techniques:
  - *Believing in Myself: What I Can Do and Say to OCB*
  - *My Toolbox*
  - *Other Things I Need or Like*
  - *Thinking Differently and Outsmarting OCB*
- Review the **Functional Behavior Assessment and Intervention (FBAI) Summary Form** distributed in the Caregiver Module as appropriate.
- Use the completed sheets on coping techniques to decide as a team what should be added.
- Last, fill out the rewards by referring to the completed **Rewarding Yourself** and **Small and Big Rewards** worksheets or choosing from the

options on the completed **Stepping It Up: Completing My Exposures** sheet from last week.

Note: At this point, children will complete Break and Snack (10 Min.) and Social Skills Activity: Picture Prep (15 Min.) while Caregivers complete Caregiver Module 8: Reinforcement Thinning (25 Min.)

Break and Snack

You may continue to offer snacks from the **Reinforcer Checklist** (Chapter 1, Appendix B). Allow this break period to be child-directed (e.g., a child may want to draw or attempt to initiate a game with you). You can capitalize on this time to build rapport with the children or facilitate rapport building within the group. If helpful, use a timer and give children reminders of the time remaining.

You may use this time to observe OCBs or contrive situations to collect descriptive data (if possible) using the **ABC Narrative Form** (Chapter 3, Appendix B) or you may use one of your own.

Social Skills Activity: Picture Prep

Picture Prep requires children to practice taking turns and attending to others. This is an **advanced** social skill activity (see Chapter 4 for further details).

Instructions: Ask the children what they will need to take pictures with their friends. Facilitate having the children ask their peers to take a picture together. Prompt children who are waiting for a turn to write down ideas of what they'd like to do in their pictures.

In a one-on-one setting, the child can create their picture independently, with a preferred activity (e.g., their construction project). See Chapter 4 for additional modifications.

Individualized Interventions for the Multiple Targeted OCBs

Refer to your **Cognitive Behavioral Skills Template.** If time permits, have children fill out the **OCB News** for OCBs where you think this would be helpful. Continue to fade your guidance and have the caregiver assume a more independent role. See previous sessions for an explanation of the four types of coping techniques: **Believing in Myself: What I Can Do and Say to OCB, My Toolbox, Other Things I Need or Like, Thinking Differently, and Outsmarting OCB**. Complete the **Rewarding Yourself** and **Small and Big Rewards** activities as needed.

Completing E/RP Worksheets for the Multiple Targeted OCBs

Explain to the child that it is now time to complete their homework sheet called **Stepping It Up and Completing My Exposures**. See previous sessions for a detailed explanation of how to complete each of the components. Given Caregiver Modules 7 and 8 are on Choosing and Thinning Reinforcers, attempt to have caregivers take a larger role in the selection and thinning of reinforcers and programming for OCBs at desired levels and new OCBs.

Token Exchange and Goodbyes

Complete the token exchange and have the children say goodbye to one another.

Caregiver Module 8: Reinforcement Thinning

Review and Introduction

Distribute new **Caregiver Weekly Data Forms** (Chapter 2, Appendix E). Let caregivers know to bring forward issues or challenges when tackling OCBs, or any new OCBs that arise.

Tell the caregivers that this week's module will involve continuing to fill out their child's **Stepping It Up and Completing My Exposures** worksheet for new OCBs and how to thin reinforcers.

Instruction

Explain reinforcement thinning to the caregivers. As children become more successful with using coping strategies and replacement behaviors, you can begin to thin reinforcement. This may involve gradually providing reinforcement less frequently. It may mean providing a token or a reinforcer once every two, three, or four times the child is successful at completing daily exposure steps instead of every time. It can also mean providing gradually smaller amounts of the preferred items. Some planned reinforcers (e.g., tokens) should be faded out entirely so that natural reinforcers (e.g., verbal praise) take their place. For example, consider a child who is learning to start a conversation in replacement of asking for reassurance about germs. We might begin by providing tokens or a highly preferred activity when that child is first successful in starting conversations. As they continue to be successful, we will give them tokens or a preferred item once every few times. Eventually, the tokens or preferred item can be completely faded out so that the social interaction that occurs when starting a conversation with a caregiver or another individual becomes the reinforcer.

Modeling

Give each caregiver their completed copy of the E/RP worksheet from last week. Show them how to plan for thinning reinforcement using the following example:

- Example: Decreasing handwashing duration (Children's Workbook)
  - The child has reached the goal of one minute of handwashing (the desired duration for this behavior). Collect data for one more week to ensure it remains at one minute.
  - Once the child has sustained this duration (this is known as maintenance), start providing progressively smaller reinforcers (e.g.,

providing five minutes of extra iPad time instead of ten) or deliver reinforcers less frequently (e.g., providing extra iPad time every other day instead of daily if exposure steps are met).

Rehearsal

Work together with caregivers to generate ideas about how their child's reinforcers can be thinned to more naturalistic consequences for one of their child's previous OCBs. For instance, caregivers can create a separate box on the worksheet next to the planned reinforcers and write down how each planned reinforcer will be thinned (e.g., write down five minutes of extra iPad time in the box next to the original ten minutes of extra iPad time). Alternatively, you could photocopy an extra **Stepping It Up and Completing My Exposures** worksheet and the caregivers could start from scratch.

Feedback

Provide positive and specific praise when the caregiver completes a portion of the worksheet correctly (e.g., "Those are great thinning steps!") and corrective feedback for incorrect/incomplete components (e.g., "You can probably thin reinforcement a little faster. Let's think of another option for that next step").

Scheduling Follow-Up Meetings

Review the **Functional Behavior Assessment and Intervention (FBAI) Summary Form** (Session 2, Appendix C) for the new OCB. If needed, continue to review the completed FBAI for the OCB during individualized programming. Take a few minutes to schedule follow-up meetings with caregivers to complete the FBA for the next OCB (see Chapter 3 for details). Finalize which OCB will be the focus of the upcoming session.

Chapter 14

Session 9

Revisiting Quality of Life, Wrap-Up, and Graduation

Materials

- Children's Workbook
- Flipchart/Whiteboard
- Token Board (Session 1, Appendix A)
- Tokens and grab bag of preferred items
- Activities/food items for break/snack
- Reinforcer Checklist (Chapter 1, Appendix B)
- ABC Narrative Form (Chapter 3, Appendix B)
- Picture Perfect materials, printed photos, and craft materials (e.g., popsicle sticks, glue, pencil crayons, sparkle glue, scissors)
- Cognitive Behavioral Skills Template (Session 2, Appendix A)
- Blank Caregiver Weekly Data Form (Chapter 2, Appendix E)
- Completed Graduation Certificates

Session Outline

- Homework Review (15 Min.)
- Review of Previous Work on OCBs and Further Programming (25 Min.)
- Break Snack (10 Min.)
- Social Skills Activity: Picture Perfect (15 Min.)
- Individualized Interventions for the Targeted OCBs (At the Discretion of Child and Caregiver) (35 Min.)
- Revisiting Quality of Life (10 Min.)
- Graduation (5 Min.)
- Token Exchange and Goodbyes (5 Min.)
- Caregiver Module 9: Wrap-Up, Review, and Reflection (25 Min.) – To take place during Break and Snack, and Picture Perfect

DOI: 10.4324/9781003410126-14

Pre-Session Checklist

- Arrange the environment (e.g., seating) as you feel appropriate.
- You may continue to outline the session activities on a whiteboard or flipchart.
- Have child **Token Boards** ready with prosocial behaviors written on them. Vary tokens to depict preferred pictures or stickers to maintain interest.
- Complete the **Cognitive Behavioral Skills Template** (Session 2, Appendix A) for next target OCB (if applicable).
- Prepare new **Caregiver Weekly Data Forms** (Chapter 2, Appendix E), if applicable.
- Complete the **Functional Behavior Assessment and Intervention (FBAI) Summary Form** (based on functional behavior assessment completed) for next target OCB (Session 2, Appendix C), if applicable.
- Complete the **Graduation Certificates** with each participant's name and signed by therapists.

Session Implementation

Homework Review

Review today's schedule and hand out the **Token Boards** (Session 1, Appendix A) with prosocial behaviors written on them for today's session. Have children give a brief review of progress and share their experiences with obsessive-compulsive behaviors (OCBs). Leading prompts to encourage conversation should be offered as needed.

Using the stimulus map, the **Caregiver Weekly Data Forms** (Chapter 2, Appendix E), and the completed **Stepping It Up: Completing My Exposures** sheet, discuss progress and obstacles with target OCBs, and those still requiring program modifications in this final session. Ask the question: *Should your OCBs be moved on the map?* Children will likely initiate this on their own.

Encourage practice and independence in using coping techniques in the moment to support relapse prevention. You may also have the child look at OCBs in various zones on the stimulus map and discuss setting events (or circumstances that lead to an increased likelihood of OCBs occurring). Have the child and caregiver brainstorm setting events and triggers of OCB, focusing on common setting events (e.g., a difficult transition, increased noise, deprivation of attention), and problem-solve ways to resist the urge and prevent re-emergence. Continue the discussion from last week and generate multiple examples, especially with classes of OCBs that have been worked on.

Talk to the children about how proud they should feel for all the hard work they have done. Explain to children that the workbook was not only developed to help them learn different things and keep track of their progress, but it can also serve as a valuable resource to refer to whenever they need it. In our experience, of the children and caregivers who have used this workbook in the past, those who refer to it when needed generally report success in preventing OCBs from coming back and find it to be a useful resource if new OCBs pop up!

Discuss what OCBs are left and need to be programmed for in Session 9. In some cases, children and caregivers may want to develop a complete intervention plan for an OCB that they can work on and discuss post-treatment (e.g., in a booster session). In this case, a functional behavior assessment (FBA) may be scheduled for this coming week, and this can be further discussed in Caregiver Module 9.

Suggested Criteria for Moving to the Next OCBs

Use the data (caregiver data sheets, stimulus map, E/RP worksheets) and a discussion with the caregiver and child to decide whether to program for an additional OCB in this session. Over one week, if progress is being made, you should see some movement towards desired levels on the caregiver rating sheet for individual OCBs (e.g., a rating of five to a rating of three over several days). Also, the child should show increased fluency in using the coping techniques and indicate some success in resisting OCB (which would be indicated by several successful attempts on E/RP steps and using coping techniques). The stimulus map can be used for discussion and assessing progress.

1. Minimal Progress: If the criteria are not met, the team (child, caregiver, therapist) may decide jointly to continue working on the same OCBs.
2. Good Progress: If the child has continued to make good progress on targeted OCBs and has remained at desired levels (with no need for using coping techniques) for at least one week, discontinue data collection. One week is usually not enough. It will be more likely that the child made some progress, but you encourage continued work in the 25-minute "Review of Previous Work on OCBs."

Encourage generalization to other stimuli, settings, and people as appropriate. Discuss OCBs that still need to be tackled and brainstorm useful coping techniques.

After the break and Caregiver Module, you may develop new individualized treatment plans for OCBs on the **Stepping It Up: Completing My Exposures** worksheet (at the child and caregiver's discretion).

Review of Previous Work on OCBs and Further Programming

Take this time to review the previous work on OCBs and continue programming as needed. See Session 8 for a brief review of further programming for previously targeted OCBs.

Note: At this point, children will complete Break and Snack (10 Min.) and Social Skills Activity: Picture Perfect (15 Min.) while Caregivers complete Caregiver Module 9: Wrap-Up, Review, and Reflection (25 Min.).

Break and Snack

You may continue to offer snacks from the **Reinforcer Checklist** (Chapter 1, Appendix B). You may use this time to observe OCBs or contrive situations to collect descriptive data (if possible) using the **ABC Narrative Form** (Chapter 3, Appendix B) or you may use one of your own.

Social Skills Activity: Picture Perfect

Picture Perfect requires children to reflect on what they have learned and create a memorable item they can take with them after the program ends. This is an advanced social skill activity (see Chapter 4 for further details).

Instructions: Lay the photos from the previous week out on a table. Ask the children to come up and find their photos. Then, have the children gather up any art supplies that they might need and facilitate children working on making a card for a friend/instructor, or a picture to remember the group.

In a one-on-one setting, the child may informally share and discuss their picture with the therapist or caregivers. See Chapter 4 for additional modifications.

Individualized Interventions for the Targeted OCBs
(At the Discretion of Child and Caregiver)

Refer to your **Cognitive Behavioral Skills Template**. If time permits, have children fill out the **OCB News** for OCBs where you think this would be helpful. See previous sessions for an explanation of the four types of coping techniques: **Believing in Myself: What I Can Do and Say to OCB, My Toolbox, Other Things I Need or Like, Thinking Differently, and Outsmarting OCB**. Complete the **Rewarding Yourself** and **Small and Big Rewards** activities as needed.

Completing E/RP Worksheets for the Targeted OCBs

Explain to the child that it is now time to complete their homework sheet called **Stepping It Up and Completing My Exposures**. See previous sessions for a detailed explanation of how to complete each component.

Revisiting Quality of Life

Take a final visit back to Session 5 and the Quality of Life circle. You may reflect on things like how many more favorite things and people can be seen (if this is the case). If preferred things and people are still covered, what are the next steps (e.g., booster sessions)? For each child, focus on their progress and recognize that this may vary across participants. Discuss where gains were made (big and small) and how this relates to OCBs being less interfering and increases in their quality of life. Bring the conversation back to how proud they should be for being brave and believing in themselves. Encourage active participation from children and caregivers.

Graduation

Congratulate each child for being brave and taking part in Fb-CBT. Give a final reminder to review their workbooks if OCB pops back into their life again. Provide certificates of completion.

Token Exchange and Goodbyes

Complete the token exchange and have the children say goodbye to one another.

Caregiver Module 9: Wrap-Up, Review, and Reflection

Review and Introduction

Tell the caregivers that this week's module will focus on addressing any outstanding questions, reviewing what caregivers have learned during past modules, and reflecting on relapse prevention.

Because this is the last week, the module format will be flexible and discussion-based rather than following the standard Behavioral Skills Training model.

Discussion

Relapse Prevention

Tell caregivers to encourage their children to continue practicing coping techniques "in the moment" and intermittently throughout the day for multiple OCBs. Continue exploring triggers and setting events for past and current OCBs. Encourage caregivers to build on the discussion that took place in the session.

Reflect on the Treatment Process

Have caregivers reflect on the past nine sessions. You could choose to have an open-ended discussion now or ask them specific questions to generate discussion. Some examples are as follows:

- Identify some potential barriers to your child's OCB maintenance.
  - Brainstorm times and/or circumstances when you anticipate your child's OCBs will arise in the future.
  - What are some barriers to implementing the function-based strategies you learned over the past nine sessions?

- Identify strategies for overcoming these barriers, preventing re-emergence, and maintaining their child's success.
  - Encourage your child to look back to the Children's Workbook whenever they feel the urge to complete a compulsion.

Finally, caregivers should be asked if they have questions not yet addressed.

Booster Sessions

During the session, some children may have created individualized pro-gram plans for new OCBs. In these cases, booster sessions should be arranged as required.

Index